W.E.T.s 4 VETS®

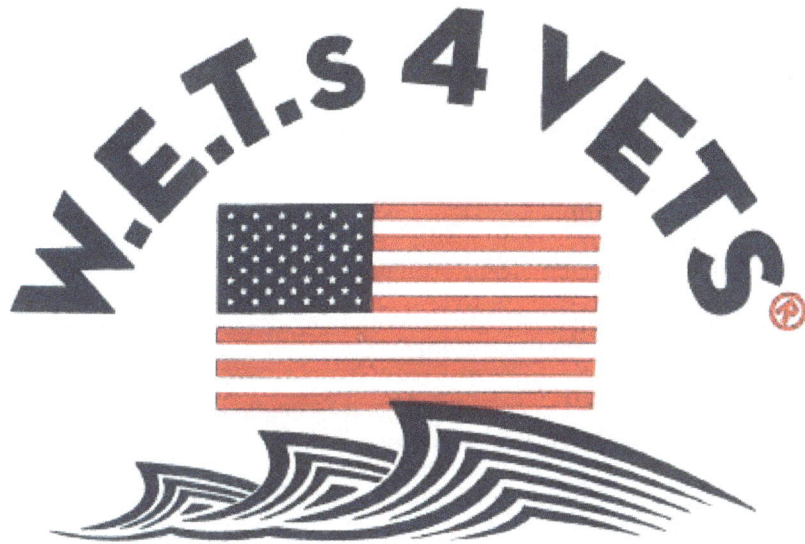

An instructional manual for veterans acclimating to civilian life

First Printing: September 2022

Other Books by Jane Katz

1. Swimming for Total Fitness, A Complete Program for Swimming Stronger, Faster, and Better, Broadway Books/Random House, NY, updated 2005

2. Exercícios Aquáticos na Gravidez (Portuguese). Sao Paulo, Brazil, 2005.

3. Natación Para Todos (swimming for Everyone, in Spanish), Tutor, Madrid, Spain, 1995, 2004.

4. Your Water Workout: No-Impact Aerobic and Strength Training From Yoga, Pilates, Tai Chi, and More. Broadway Books, New York, NY, 2003.

5. Ejercicios en el Agua para todos (Exercises in the Water for Everyone), Tutor, Madrid, 2000.

6. Water Fitness During Your Pregnancy (translated into Korean), 1999.

7. The New W.E.T. Workout ® (Water Exercise Techniques). Facts on File, New York, 1996.

8. The All-American Aquatic Handbook: Your Passport to Lifetime Fitness, Allyn & Bacon, Boston, 1996

9. The Aquatic Handbook for Lifetime Fitness, Allyn & Bacon, Boston, 1996.

10. Water Fitness During Your Pregnancy, Human Kinetics, Champaign, IL, 1995.

11. Swimming for Total Fitness, updated (with Nancy P. Bruning), Doubleday, New York, 1993

12. Swim 30 Laps in 30 Days: A World Master's Program for Swimming Farther, Faster and Better Putnam, New York, NY, 1991

13. Fitness Works! ™, A Blueprint for Lifelong Fitness, Leisure Press, Champaign, IL, 1988.

14. The W.E.T. Workout ® (Water Exercise Techniques). Facts on File, New York, 1985.

15. Swim Through Your Pregnancy. Doubleday, New York, NY, 1983.

16. Swimming for Total Fitness: A Progressive Aerobic Program (with Nancy P. Bruning), Doubleday, New York, NY, 1981.

Editor: Dr. Tim Johnson

Publisher: Global Aquatics
               www.globalaquatics.com

W.E.T.s 4 VETS ™ Register Trademark. No. 4,957,351 Registered: May 10, 2016.

ISBN 978-1-7340463-0-4

Dedication

To the many veterans that I have met to whom we owe our freedom, thank you. To my late father, Professor Leon Katz, and late husband Herbert Erlanger, M.D., were both veterans. Dr. Jane Katz lead the Great American Workout on the White House lawn in 1990 when General Colin Powell, an eventual United States Secretary of State, made an appearance. Both are graduates of City College of NY and are Townsend Harris Medal honoree for outstanding CCNY Alumnus.

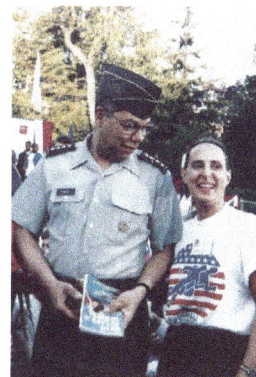

Acknowledgements

The author would like to extent her gratitude to the following persons who contributed their time, material or comments toward this new water exercise book for veterans: Susy Mendes and her research staff at John Jay College, Welby Alcantara, Capt. Ricard Pusateri, Marine Lt. Mark McNaughton, enlisted Army veterans Jonathan Martinez and Cinttia Moreno, and to many more veterans who participated in this program. To the civilian students who participated, I say thank you. Finally, a special thank you to Dr. Timothy Johnson for helping prepare and edit the manuscript.

Water is the great equalizer, it works for every body, and it is democratic.
Dr. Jane Katz, Ed.D.

Contents

Preface

How did W.E.T.s 4 VETS® begin? After a quarter of a century teaching aquatics at Bronx Community College, Dr. Katz transferred to John Jay College of Criminal Justice. John Jay specializes in training New York's uniformed services employees. While at John Jay, Dr. Katz noticed students taken her swimming classes were not traditional college students. They were veterans. Their new task was to integrate all they have learned and experienced in the military service with civilian life.

For many returning veterans, college is a viable option for realizing their goals in civilian life. John Jay's specialization in Criminal Justice attracts many students already working in the New York Police and Fire Departments, and NYC Correctional system. The college encourages returning veterans and others from structured environments to seek out careers in law enforcement. But so many things have changed; the veterans themselves are different than before their military service, the world is different, and the school environment is different. How could the college help them adapt?

Often veterans, whether students or not, struggle with stress, depression, and lack of physical activity which are symptoms of post-traumatic stress disorder (PTSD). Dr. Katz invited a few veterans to visit her swim classes and the number grew by word of mouth. The numbers grew to the extent that she organized a non-credit swim class during student activities hours to bring veterans and civilian students together. The hope was that in a non-academic setting, students can get to know, learn from, and trust each other in an aquatic environment. From this, the W.E.T.s 4 VETS® program began in 2012.

W.E.T.s® (Water Exercise Techniques) and swimming skills are often strenuous and require good health for participation. Always consult your physician before beginning any exercise program. This general information is not intended to diagnose any medical condition. Make an appointment with your healthcare provider to participate in the W.E.T.s 4 VETS® program. If you experience any pain or difficulty with these exercises, stop and make an appointment with your physician.

Chapter 1 Introduction

W.E.T.s 4 VETS® is an approach that addresses several social needs: introduction to an aquatic environment, improving participant fitness level and when combined with veterans it helps heal PTSD symptoms, and gives veterans a means to adapt to civilian life. Using a holistic approach, veterans are welcomed back to civilian life with equanimity through use of the buddy system while learning fitness and aquatic skills. This provides an opportunity for veterans to adjust to civilian life through the sharing of a common experience with civilians. W.E.T.s 4 VETS® explores this method for teaching fitness and swimming and gives the swim community a role in bring aquatic justice to everyone.

This instruction manual begins with an introduction to the teaching Methodology for this program. Holistic methods are employed to encompasses the mind, body, and spirit. The mind is addressed in understanding the lessons working within the buddy system, the body is addressed through immersion in the water, and the spirit in the commitment to accomplish the assigned exercises and activities. This is followed by the discussion of the Immersion experience which means more than just entering the water and takes into its scope the meaning of a swim community as a metaphor for the human condition. Program components are listed

Sample Lessons are divided into two parts: fitness and swimming. Both are covered in each session according to the instructors choosing to meet the needs of the participants. There is a brief discussion of what physical fitness is and the training effect. The lessons provide passive and active exercises for participants to experience the healing power of water. They begin with warm-up and warm-down exercises that are familiar to everyone as they are stretching exercises adapted for use in the aquatic environment. These 24 exercises are provided in brief. Fuller explanations of the exercises are provided in *The New WET Workout*, another of the author's books. Then the Suggested Lessons progress into swim instructions.

The buddy system is explained in depth in the swim lessons. Instructions provide a step by step understanding of how the buddy system works with the instruction of swimming. The goal for each lesson and a fun component is included in the instructions. The 15 suggested swim lessons are not all encompassing which provide subsequent certified instructors using the W.E.T.s 4 VETS® Instructional Manual the opportunity to bring their own creativity to the program.

The chapter on PTSD looks at information on the current knowledge of this injury with links for additional study. Participants graduate from the course with the skills necessary to continue (?) to practice their fitness, improve their swimming and continue building social connection in the larger community. In this chapter is a section on how W.E.T.s 4 VETS® presents students with opportunities for leadership roles, improved self-confidence, and lifelong learning skills.

A final summary is provided so that readers and participants can verify their experience. There are anonymous student testimonials about how the W.E.T.s 4 VETS® program has affected their lives. Examples of press coverage for the program are presented and biographical details are provided about the author. A paper presented by the author at the Pentagon on fitness is included.

The Appendix has convenient form sheets useful for participants. There are sample sign-in sheets and a sample medical waiver.

1.1   Immersion

The military experiences of veterans are unique to their group. In W.E.T.s 4 VETS® they have the opportunity for a shared experience of interacting with water and learning aquatic skills together. This program introduces veterans and civilians to the water space using the buddy system. In the context of learning to swim, they immerse themselves in an aquatic activity.

As the veterans and civilians learn and practice aquatics skills together, they gain in self-confidence as they trust what they have learned. They feel good about themselves and gain confident because they are now standing, floating, and swimming in a pool along with their buddies. They get immediate positive feedback as they learn to swim safely.

The medium of the water itself has a role in this methodology. When you swim you are immersed in a liquid which changes your balance and weight, giving you power and freedom of movement but at the same time a feeling of helplessness for the novice swimmer. They are entering a world unlike other activities. Your mind takes heed; these are the emotional levels through which learning is acquired.

Veterans have been trained to complete goals as a team. In the military, it is called "got your back." In the water, it is the same mindset; in the pool, students take on joint assignments and find ways to assist each other to reach their aquatic goals. For civilians who join them this will be a new experience.

Although the veterans of the 21st century face many challenges, one advantage they now have is the support of their communities to help their re-entry. Local institutions are actively exploring ways to be of service to men and women who have served our country. Aquatic facilities, both public and private, have an opportunity to support veterans by organizing W.E.T.S 4 VETS® programs in their own communities. Input from local veterans can provide ideas of what is needed and helpful. Educational institutions can participate by hosting an 'open-house' family day and other events for veterans.

1.2   Methodology

A holistic teaching method is used, encompassing mind, body and spirit.   The water environment provides a challenge to the participants of equal difficulty that lets the participants explore their inner self while facing what for them is an unknown.   In this striving to achieve aquatic mastery, they learn to relax and find strength within themselves to trust others. By setting swim goals for the students mixed with fun, the students gain self-confidence as they become more relaxed and comfortable in the water and with each other. This is a learning outcome that touches on the emotional self of students when they discover the enjoyment of the challenge, the fun of achieving the goals set out for them. and celebrate their transitioning from beginner to a better swimmer with each task.   The trust the swimmers learn from the buddy system comes from two persons helping each other complete the goals of the program.   This is extended to a community lesson by rotation of partners for each task.   This adaption of the buddy system is translated from the military "got-your-back" mind-set.   In this case, participants literally help support their swim partner's back when learning to float as they improve their social skills essential for lifelong friendships.

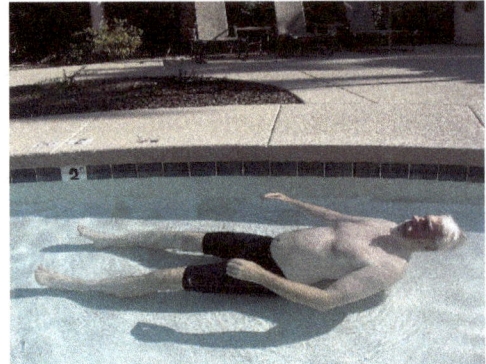

W.E.T.s 4 VETS® sessions consist of ten to twenty participants made up from the college's diverse and inclusive student body.   They meet weekly for ten weeks over the course of a semester at the John Jay College pool during the student's community time for this non-credit activity.   The group includes veterans and non-veterans.   Before the session begins, they may drink some water, eat some fruit, or take a bite of a power bar in the locker room or on the pool deck during their meet and greet period.   A typical W.E.T.S 4 VETS® workout begins with a 5 to 10 minutes warm-up followed by a main set of lessons lasting approximately 30 minutes. Instead of laps, the buddies engage in completing and mastering tasks as a group.   With each new task the buddies rotate partners as they build social skills as well as acquire aquatic skills. The warm-down consists of a 5-minute fun game of water volleyball using several beach balls. Nourishment afterwards is encouraged for the group.

1.3 Warmups Are Important

Your W.E.T.S 4 VETS workout begins with a warmup on the pool deck and continues into the pool. Several dry land stretches are simple to do and don't take long. Stretching exercises will help improve flexibility of joints and warm up the muscles. The next step is to acclimate yourself to the water temperature. Bend down to splash some water on yourself; or kneel, squat, sit on the pool edge. The idea is to begin immersing yourself in the water. If there are steps or a ladder, use those mean of accessing the water. Begin bobbing is another method immerse yourself and it gets your legs working. The body will adjust gradually to the water temperature and your ability to tolerate this change is through activity. If you can safely get to deeper water where you can stand, begin walking on the pool bottom. Swimmers will begin swimming before that depth. Once there, walk or jog in place swing or pumping your arms just like you would on land. Having water shoes on will make these exercises more comfortable if the pool surface is rough. Once you are in the water, your weight will be quite a bit less, making bad knees happy you've joined W.E.T.S 4 VETS.

Nearly any exercise you can do while standing on land you can do in the water. The advantages are the water resistance and reduce weight on your lower extremities and back. Some people will be able to do exercise that would be difficult for them execute on land. Examples of land exercises that are exactly same in the water are: head turns, shoulder rolls, twist that rotate at the waist, triceps and shoulder stretches, overhead stretch, runner leg stretch (hamstrings), and quadricep stretches.

Since both buddies are doing the same or different warm up exercises the extent of the buddy system is to allow a conversation to begin or continue. This program encourages participants to learn about themselves, unlike a water exercise class where everybody changes exercises on cue from the instructor. If you need less or more of one or another exercise, feel free to engage your self-determination if it doesn't interrupt the session—let your buddy know. Also, if you need more help or additional instruction, let your instructor know.

To make warm-ups/downs an activity that people enjoy, various exercises can be strung together with music.

1.4   Comparison with land exercises

Aquatic equipment has designated uses but when used for fitness, the water resistance is much stronger than it is on land making them a tool for fitness. An example is a kickboard. A kickboard movement on land is unrestricted by how the board is moved; but try moving the board broadside to the water and you'll have considerable trouble. It becomes a large awkward paddle. Pressing a kickboard straight down to submerge it will exercise the triceps using resistance due to the board's buoyance which is an easier exercise than pushups. Lifting a kickboard out of the water when it is flat to the water surface is not too difficult when done slowly…exercising the biceps, deltoids, and pectorals. Lifting it out of the water creates a waterfall. Other pieces of aquatic equipment like barbells*, noodles, or hand paddles can be used for resistance training for therapy or relaxed exercise through floatation.

Jumping jacks on land are easy, but in the water, they add lateral resistance to leg movement that makes this exercise more useful in overall conditioning. Fins are useless on land except as part of a clown costume but adds power and speed to swimming. A pull-buoy is a small floatation device shaped so that it can be placed between your legs for support of the legs while swimming and has other uses to take advantage of its floatation characteristics. There are belts made with floatation to allow individuals to walk/run through deep water as if they were on land.

1.5   What is Physical Fitness?

Physical fitness is the ability of the body to function at an optimum level in emergency situations as well as everyday living. Strength, muscular endurance, flexibility, body composition, motor coordination, and cardiovascular efficiency are the basic components of physical fitness. All these components can be improved by doing the W.E.T.s 4 VETS program, which exercises your heart and lungs over a sustained period of time.

Strength is the capacity of a muscle to exert force against a resistance. Endurance allows the muscle to repeatedly exert a force or maintain static contraction over time. Flexibility is the range of motion of a specific joint and its corresponding muscle group. Body composition refers to the relative amounts of muscle, bone, and fat in a body. Motor coordination combined with skill are one's athletic ability, a combination of innate ability and practice.

Cardiovascular efficiency is one of the most important components of physical fitness. It is the capacity of your heart and lungs to function efficiently in order to bring oxygen to the tissues and remove waste products from the body. This component can be developed by the training effect.

1.5.1 The Training Effect

The training effect began with the ancient Greek wrestler, Milo, who carried a calf around on his shoulders for his training. As the calf grew, Milo grew stronger and stronger. This illustrates the principle of progressive overload and how the body learns to adapt to increased demands of work. To apply progressive overload in your W.E.T.s 4 VETS program, you can exercise in a progressive fashion so that your body is better able to handle the stresses and strains of everyday living. Your blood vessels increase in number and your heart, like other muscles, becomes stronger. The skeletal muscle fibers, when exercised, become larger and stronger. In addition, they stretch and become more flexible! Additional material on this topic is presented in the Appendix, National Conference on Military Physical Fitness.

1.5.2 The FIT principle:

Dr. Jane Katz call this the FIT principle of the training effect:

Frequency—increase the number of workouts per week.

Intensity—Increase and vary intensity with the resistance equipment.

Time—Increase the time of the main set.

A muscular, trimmed and toned athlete certainly looks fit but water exercise trains the whole body including the heart. The idea of the FIT athlete doesn't need to bulk up but has aerobic energy to go the distance.

1.5.3   Pulse Check

During your W.E.T.s 4 VETS program or whenever you exercise, pause to take your pulse by gently placing your index finger on your wrist or on either side of your neck at the carotid artery. Count the beats for six seconds and multiply by ten (add a zero to the number) to determine an approximate number of beats per minute. Your pulse rate gives you your heart rate (HR). Your Training Heart Rate (THR) is the number of beats per minute that you can train continuously. The THR is 60-85% of your Maximum Heart Rate (MHR).

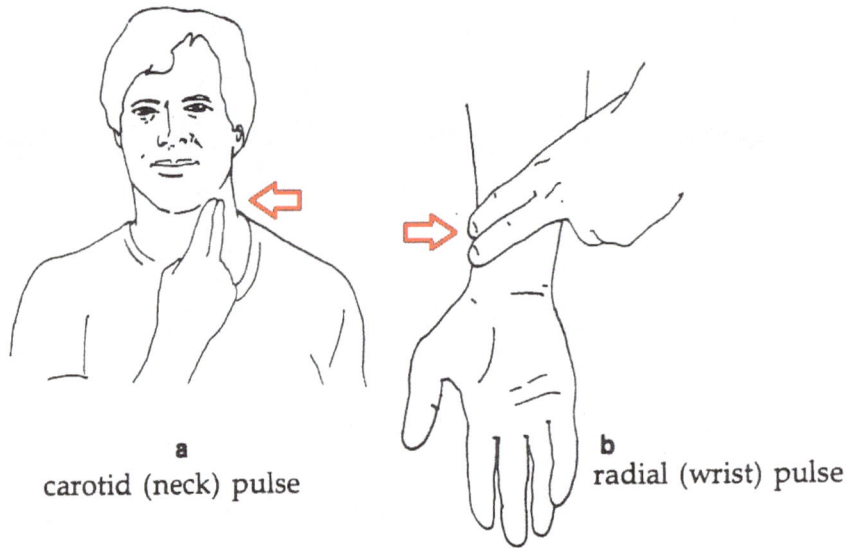

a
carotid (neck) pulse

b
radial (wrist) pulse

Figure 1 How to check your 6-second pulse rate

Your Pulse/Heart Rate Chart to collect your pulse/heart data:

Week	Date	Warm-up	Main Set	Cool down	Comments

Your pulse rate is multiplied by 10 is you used a timing interval of six seconds or by six if you used a ten second interval to determine your Heart Rate. In the Appendix, there is a full page THR Chart for your record keeping.

1.5.4   The Heart Rate Aquatic Workout

Using your pulse rate, a workout can be planned that will exercises your body without excessive stress. See the Aquatic Workout Program you design for yourself found in the Appendix. Figure 2 below shows how your pulse reveals changes to your Training Heart Rate during exercises.

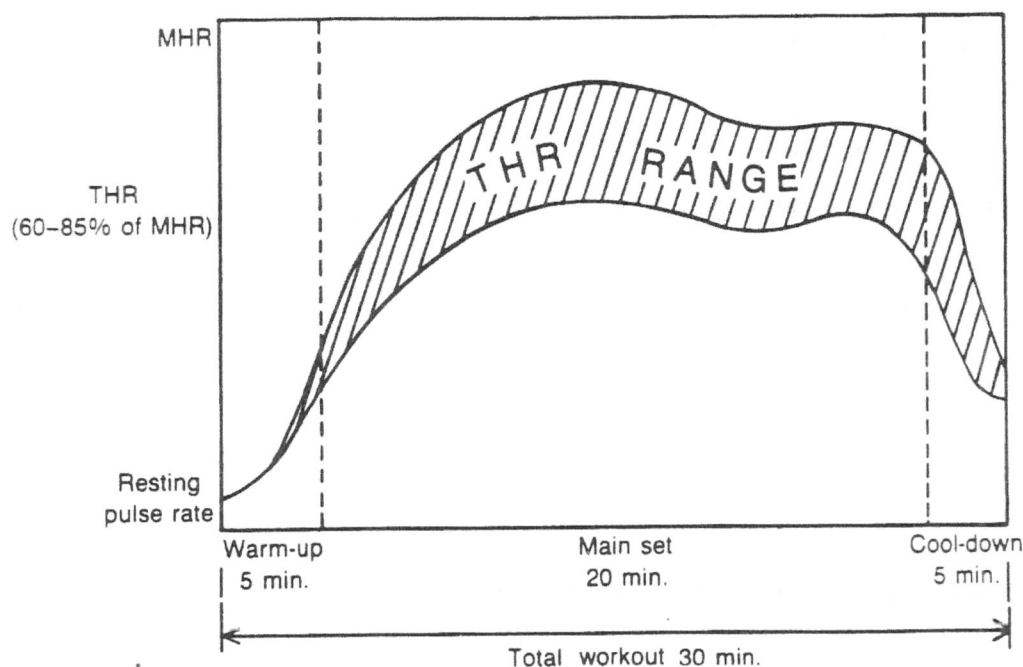

Figure 2 THR Range

With your workout planned, begin the workout by taking your baseline pulse before your warm-up. When you have finish with your warm-up, take another pulse check. During your workout, between sets of exercises, take your pulse. When your main set of exercises are completed and before beginning your cool-down, take your pulse. Finally, when you are finished with your cool-down, take a final pulse count. Your own THR Range graph can be filled out with your personal information. Over time, you will see how consist you exercise and make changes as needed.

These are a lot of numbers to remember so having some method to record the pulse counts for the Pulse Rate Chart would be handy. Currently, Fitbit and Apple watch do not work while swimming.

1.6   W.E.T.s 4 VETS program components

1.   Weekly meetings of approximately a dozen participants for twelve weeks.

2.   Participants include veterans and non-veterans.

3.   This is a non-competitive, communal, aquatic experience with social, physical and emotional aspects.

4.   The program is based on the buddy system.

    a.   At poolside, participants are paired up. Names and greetings exchanged.

    b.   Participants switch off to a different buddy for each exercise.

5.   The fun and fitness are integrated in the lessons.

6.   Providing snacks or light lunch after the session is encouraged to build community.

7.   Every session ends with a FUN water volleyball game!

8.   Music poolside at a background sound level is allowed.

1.6.1   Traditional swim equipment

Kickboards—waterfalls/ocean waves/kicking

Pull buoys—underwater tennis (swishing)/boxing (pulling & pushing) while stationary

Hand paddles—swimming skills

Swim fins—stretching/kicking assist

Noodles—floating assistance/lane markers/water limbo/challenge courses

Swim bars floats—variety of stretching exercises for warm up/celebrations/floating

1.6.2   Aquatic events

Coney Island Splash—kickboard assisted splashing and high-five greeting

Aqua Steps—in water walking/steps/running/hopping/skipping

Aqua Dancing—boogie down/water dancing to music

Buddy fun relays—use to extend range of swimmers across the pool's width (short length)

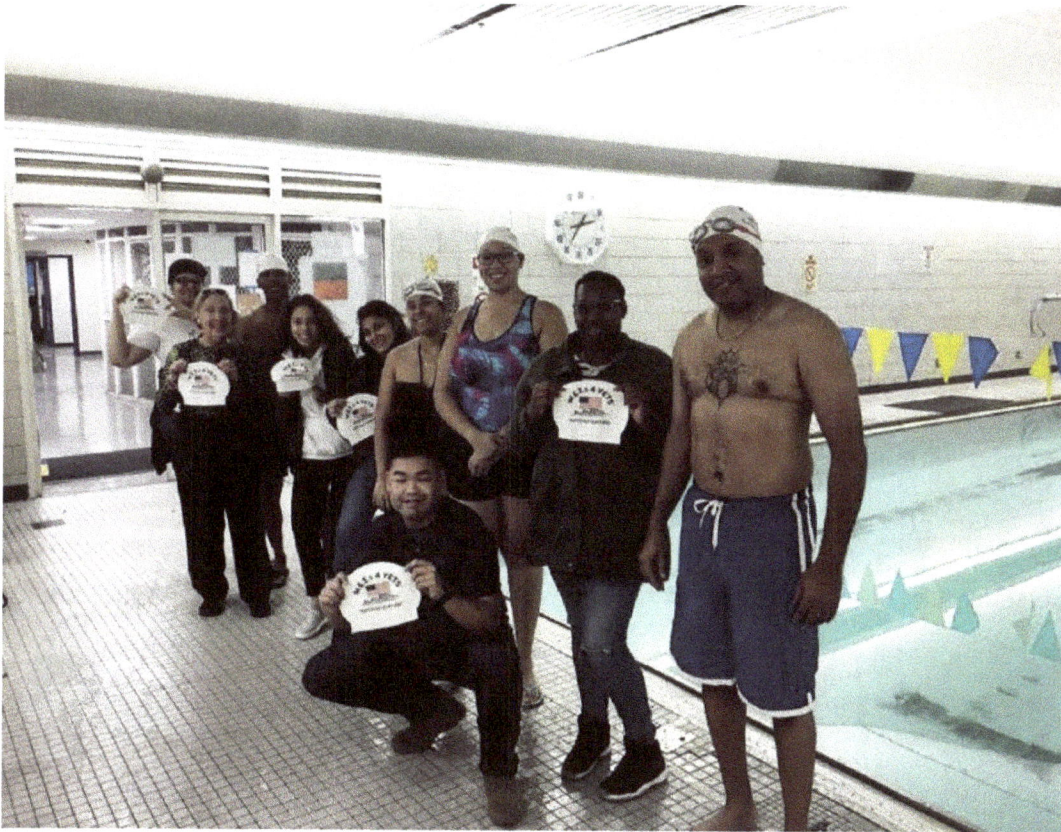

Figure 3 Typical W.E.T.s 4 VETS® participants with Dr. Jane Katz, 2nd from left

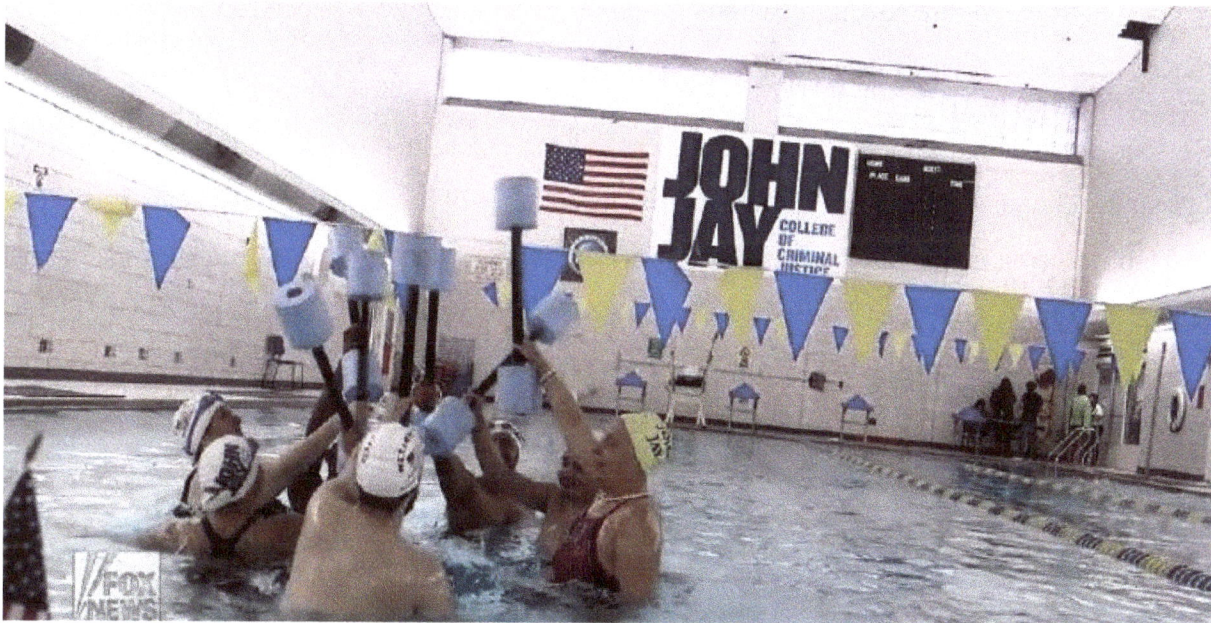

Figure 4 High 5's exercise celebration using swim bar floats

Chapter 2 Aquatic Fitness

In the W.E.T.s 4 VETS program, the basics of swimming are taught using ingenuity and a supportive approach for training with a swim buddy. The following are traditional exercises created for the W.E.T.s 4 VETS® program. After the exercise is explained and demonstrated the challenge is to have the buddies help each other accomplish the task. The exercises are by no means inclusive of all lessons but suggestive of the manner of instruction for a lesson.

2.1 Instruction mode

In a traditional setting, the novice or higher-level swimmers line up along the edge of the pool in or out of the water to hear and observer the instructor's demonstration. Then individually the students enter the water to replicate the skill with the instructor(s) by their side to observe and assist. Usually, all the students are at the same skill level (beginner) and there is one instructor for several students.

With W.E.T.s 4 VETS® instructions, most students are adults with varying aquatic skill levels. Their advantage is they can safely stand up in water depths than can range from their mid-section to chest high. Some are adequate swimmers and other may have experienced a traumatic episode that has created a fear of the water.

Lessons begin with the buddies in the water and the instructor. Instruction frequently begins with one student buddied up with the instructor. The instructor will be the active buddy and the student is the observer/assisting buddy. The instructor demonstrates what should be done in this lesson adding narrative as needed. The buddies then switch roles with the instructor becoming the observer/assisting buddy. During this time, the instructor is playing the part of the observing/assisting buddy and assisting as needed for active buddy. The instructor asks if there are any question and then for everyone to begin the lesson. The instructor then rotates around to assist students in mastering this lesson.

Remember to hydrate

2.2   Water Exercise Techniques (W.E.T.s)

The sessions begin after signing in on the pool deck where the participants select a buddy before entering the water. Since the goal is to meet and work with everyone in the class over time, who is selected as a buddy is important but as the class progresses, eventually everyone becomes your buddy. Names are exchanged, a conversation begins, then it's time to begin the first lesson.

> For safety, whenever you enter a pool area, look for water depth signage so you know the water depth before you go begin. For this lesson, you will want to be at the shallow end of the

The buddies take positions along the pool deck sitting with their feet in the water. Acclimating to the water temperature could involve splashing water in your face. Sit with your legs extended, knees straight, and feet in the water. Hands are on the deck for support. This exercise teaches you the flutter kick before entering the water. The flutter kick begins by straightening your feet and alternately moving your legs up and down brushing your big toes against one another. The feet should be going as far underwater as they are above the water. You are looking for a little splashing at a moderate speed. Your instructor will demonstrate the flutter kick for you.

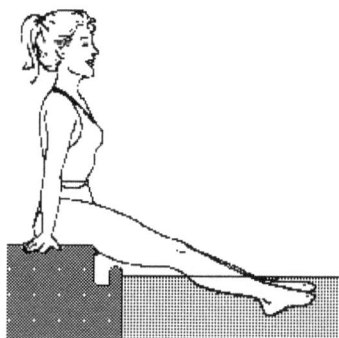

Figure 5 Sitting on pool deck with feet in the water

Entering the water is the next task. There are a variety of ways to accomplish this: using a zero entry that slopes down into the water as you would at the ocean or climbing down a pool ladder. If there are no steps, a gradual approach that works on all pools is to sit on the edge of the pool at the shallow end with your feet in the water. Rotate your body to one side placing both hands on the pool deck on that side of your body. Completely the turn supporting yourself with your shoulders as you gradually allow yourself to slide down until your feet touch the bottom. If you are hesitant, ask your instructor for assistance.

2.3   Sample Warm-up/Cool-down Exercises

When you enter the pool desk, hopefully you've taken a shower beforehand, dip your toes into the water to check the water temperature of the pool. The water depth should be between the chin to your midsection. Start with warm-up exercises which also double as cool-down exercises at the end of your workout. While you warm up, have fun and meet some new buddies that you'll be exercising with while you experience the W.E.T.s 4 VETS program. Before we take the plunge, check your pulse (section 1.5.3) for a pre-exercise baseline to compare before, during, and after your program workout ends. We often finish the W.E.T.s 4 VETS exercises with a beach ball where the receiver of the ball announces their name with everyone repeating the name.

When you wake up in the morning we usually stretch. One of them is called a triceps stretch. Put your arms are over your head maybe you need your other arm to help your elbow become as vertical as possible to help stretch your shoulder your back and let's get started once you do one side guess what we do the other as well let's repeat the entire right and left sides twice good job you're on your way.

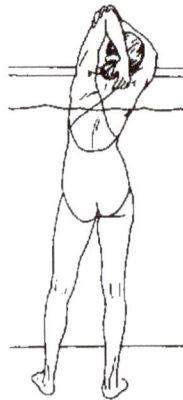

Figure 6 Triceps stretch

Remember to hydrate

The cross-chest stretch is something that we do during the day. One arm is extended across your chest just below your chin. The opposite hand helps to just gently bring your elbow of your extended arm to a comfortable position and held while you tension and stretch your shoulders while you inhale. Use the supporting hand to reposition your arm and shoulder a bit more while you exhale. Do the same on the other side. If you notice pain, ease up. More sets of this exercise can be done. You can take your pulse and check your pulse at the end of each exercise.

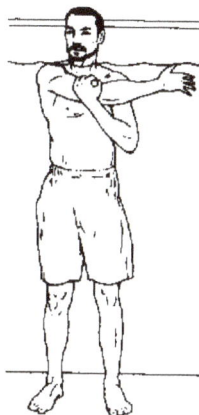

Figure 7 Cross chest stretch

Perhaps you did the standing wall stretch already this morning it's a great exercise in the water so face your right side to the edge of the pool extend your right arm and keep your body as vertical as possible and press with your hand toward the edge of the pool take two or three breaths and then stand up and turn around and repeat on the other side.

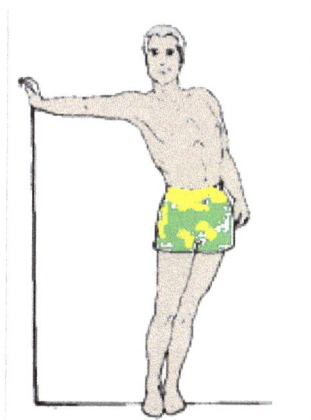

Figure 8 Standing stretch

The Quadriceps stretch occurs when standing in chest-deep water. You can hold onto the wall with one hand to steady yourself. The free hand grasps and holds your foot. Stretched and tension your upper leg as you try to straighten the leg. Try to keep your knees together. When you finish one side, rotate to the opposite side so your other leg gets exercised as well. This stretch is a very important before exercising for almost every sport.

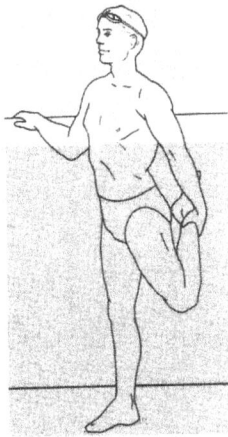

Figure 9 Runner Quad stretch

Your next exercise is the Pike body stretch. In the example shown below, you hold onto the gutter and place your legs on the pool wall. You squat pulling your chest in at the same time. Then you extend your legs outward relaxing the arms in the stretch portion of the exercise. You don't have to do it fast. This is another position you can use to stretch your Achilles tendons. As you extend your legs, try to straighten them at the knees. Your feet should be flat against the wall so that your knees control the stretch. Hold the position for three to five seconds then relax bring your feet back down to the bottom of the pool.

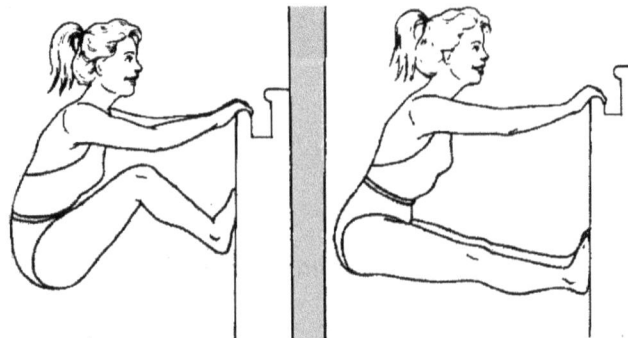

Figure 10 Pike body stretch

The Aqua Lunge is an excellent end of workout exercise as well as a warmup. Face the wall with your hands holding onto the gutter about shoulder-length apart. Position your legs so they are on the pool wall about 3 feet apart with knees slightly bent for comfort. You will then rock your body by straightening one leg, folding the other to absorb the stretch then switch to straighten the other leg. Hold the stretch for three to five seconds, slowly return to center, and then repeat on the other side. Be sure not to overdo it keeping within your comfort level.

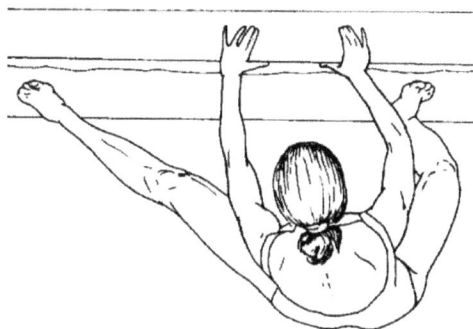

Figure 11 Aqua Lunge with left leg stretched

The Leg Lift works your abdominal muscles exercising your core body area. In the water you position yourself by holding onto the wall with your hands, arms extended. Place your upper back against the pool wall. Extend your legs under water along the water surface. Bend the knees as you draw them toward the upper body using your abdominal muscles, then extend your legs outward again. This is similar to a sit-up where your legs are held in position on a mat and your upper body raises up to meet the knees. As a water exercise, you should find it easier as you are not lifting as much weight. For extra support, using the corner of the pool will help.

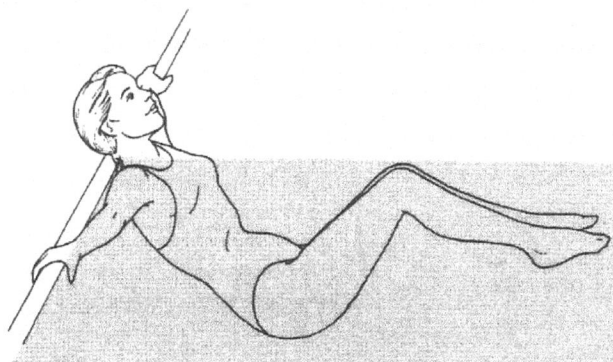

Figure 12 Leg lifts

The Calf Stretch is an exercise to release a cramp in the back of your lower leg. In the water because of the buoyancy it will be easier to develop your calf muscle by putting your entire foot on the bottom of the pool hold that for five seconds and stand up and switch to the other side. If you get leg cramps often, you might consider consuming more water. It is important to hydrate before your main set. Keep a water bottle handy and refill it before and after your workout.

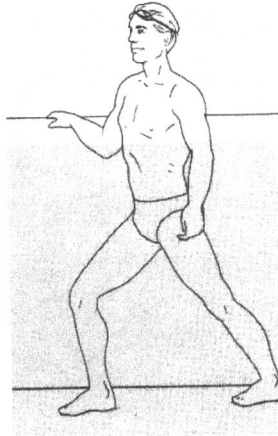

Figure 13 Runner calf stretch

The Arm Circle water exercise is good for warm-ups and cool-downs. The exercise gives you the opportunity to feel the water pressure on your hands, arms and shoulders much like a swim stroke as your arms circle underwater. Start with small circles then increase the circle size keeping your elbows straight. Your shoulders can be exercised and stressed gradually during a warm-up. This will give you a feel for the water flow by keeping your hands open.

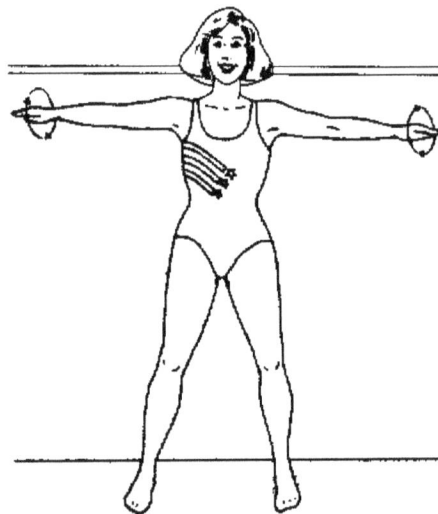

Figure 14 Arm Circles

The Overhead Stretch is performed in the water. Your arms are extended about your shoulders holding a towel held apart by tension from your arms. Hold this pose for 20 seconds, release the tension and lower your arms. Your towel may get wet. You could also bend sideways and sweep the towel overhead allowing you to bend and stretch your Lat's at the same time. Another pose is to hold one hand overhead holding the towel pulling against the other end of the towel held behind your back keeping your shoulder loose.

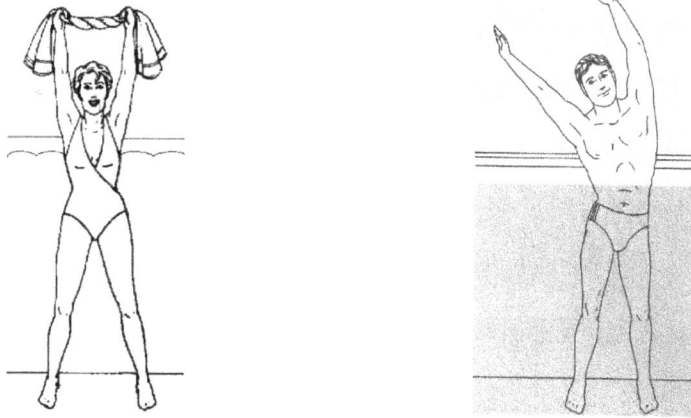

Figure 15 Overhead stretch

Your muscles of your upper body are where the strength for swimming resides as it is with boxing. Exercising in water adds resistance. Allow your body and torso to turn as you alternate your punching. Just like a boxer, you get more power in your stroke if you lean into it. A punch is similar to doing the crawl stroke entry with the opposite arm waiting to begin its punch. If you were to cup your hand as you withdraw the punch, you would be doing the dog paddle.

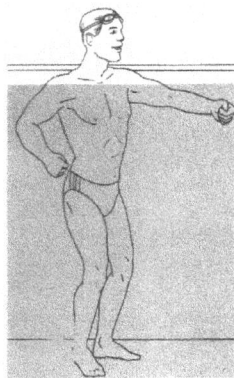

Figure 16 Boxing in water adds resistance

In addition to the boxing exercise the Golf or Tennis swing uses a pull buoy which is a very popular swimming training device used by swimmers. Grasp it in the middle of the two parts and exercise your pectoral muscles and shoulders by swinging back and forth underwater. You could do this same exercise without the pull buoys, but the equipment adds extra resistance helping your strength. The golf swing is useful for other sports as well.

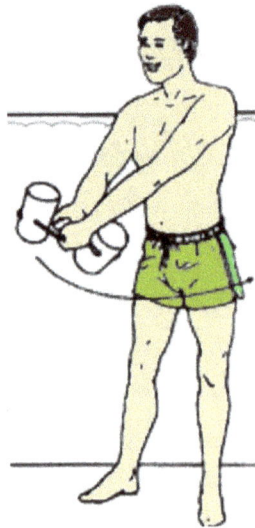

Figure 17 Golf swing

The Water Push/Pull is a basic and important exercise to warm up for your main set and cool down. Stand with one arm forward and the other behind you, swing the arms so one arm pulls water behind you and the opposite hand is drawn forward through the water for the next pull. Start a slow comfortable water walk perhaps in shallow water from one side to the other Once you establish your alternating arm motion keeping the arm relatively straight your thumbs can pass close by brushing the side of your body as you walk.

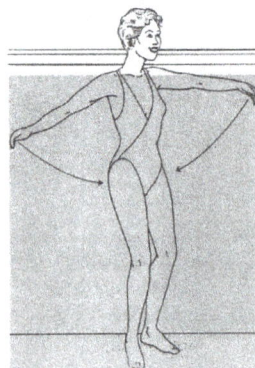

Figure 18 Water Push/Pull

Aqua Jogging is a comfortable exercise in the water an allows you to move around the pool. As the name implies, this is a slightly different accented version of water walking exaggerating your hands and your feet movements. Resistance can be added using paddles for strength and increased pulse rate. This exercise with a floatation belt can be practiced in deep water.

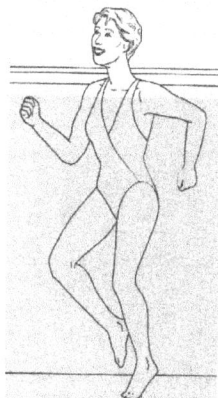

Figure 19 Aqua Jogging

The Rockette kick is a simple exercise to stretch your hamstrings in the back of your leg. You don't even need equipment. If the pool depth is graduated, this exercise is best when the water level is at your waist. Lift one leg with knee straight several time in succession then switch to the other leg. You can stand against the pool side or just hold on with one hand lifting your leg in along the pool side instead of kicking out toward the water.

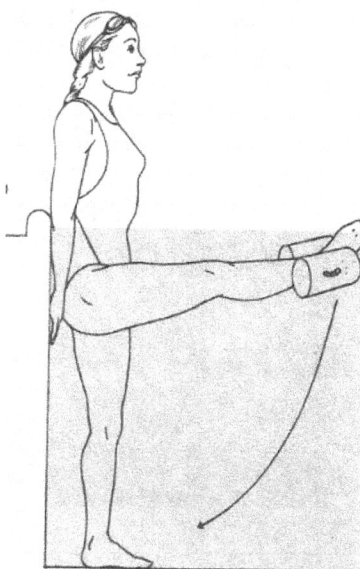

Figure 20 Rockette kick

This exercise is like another popular song: The Twist. Stand in chest deep water with hands on your hips. You twist your body from one side to the other. Your shoulders rotate with your hips, but your head stays mostly facing forward. Most strokes utilize a rotation as part of the stroke.

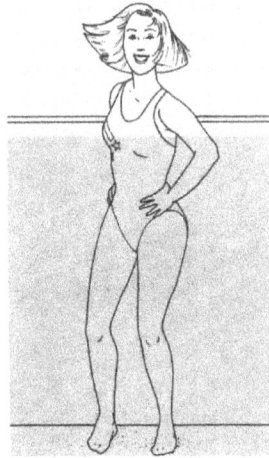

Figure 21 Trunk Twist

Exercises related to other sports are possible to do as a water exercise as rehabilitation or for strengthening muscles using water resistance. Here are a few examples:

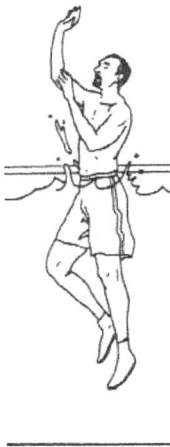 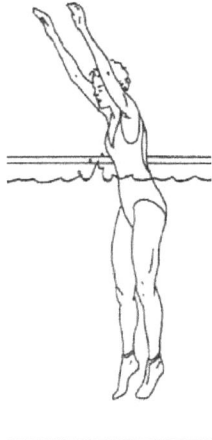 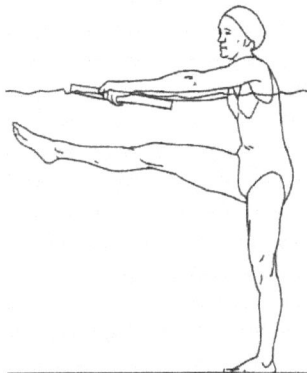 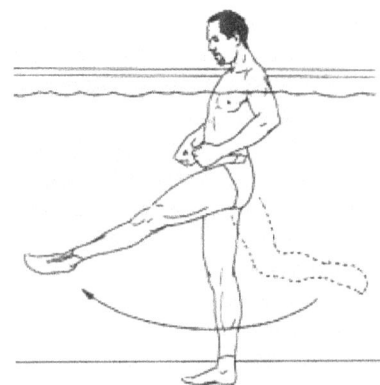

Basketball   Volleyball   Dance Kick   Soccer Kick

HAVE FUN AND PRACTICE YOUR SPORT IN THE WATER

Chapter 3 Sample Swim Skills

3.1 Show me the bubbles—bobbing and blowing bubbles

After entering the water, the buddies' line up facing the pool wall and holding onto the wall with one hand. One at a time, so the other buddy can observe, the active buddy inhales then begins to slowly exhale while submerge underwater completely. The release of air is exhaled thorough the nose and mouth together. The active buddy emerges from the water as air is exhausted. The breathing is at a normal rhythm. The goal is to have a controlled release of the air while submerged. Repeat 5 times. The next step is for the buddies to turn and face each other, grasp one another hand as if shaking their hand, then one at a time repeat this exercise. This exercise accustoms the buddies to continuous inhalation and exhalation as the face enters and leaves the water. It's also a way to relax between sets during a workout.

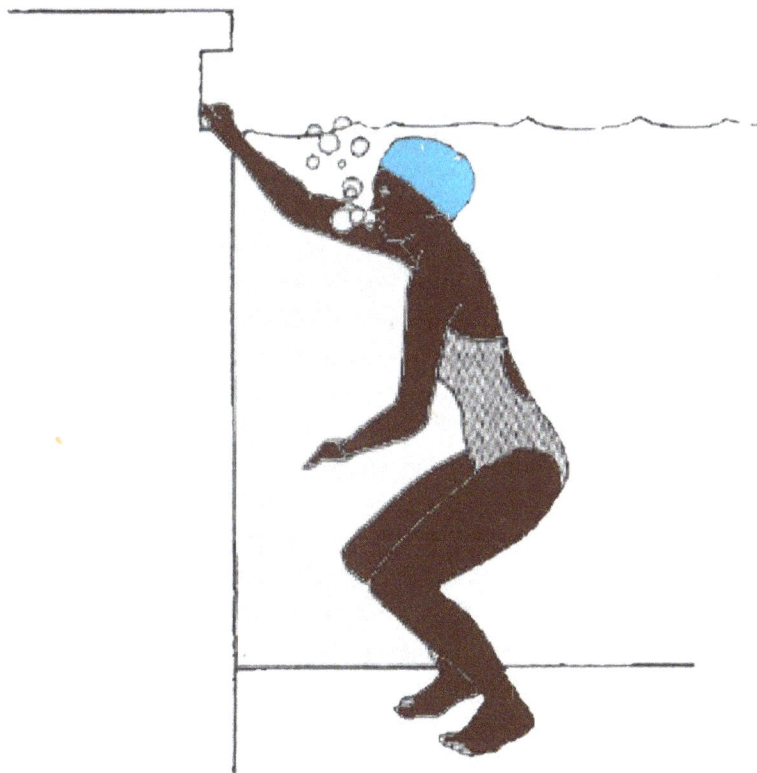

Figure 22 Bobbing and exhaling underwater while holding onto the wall.

3.2 Bobbing for safety

Your first lesson prepared you for taking your next breath by exhaling under water. The difference with this exercise and the previous is you are not holding onto the side of the pool. Take a step back from the wall, inhale, and exhale under the water by submerging. What is the same is you can jump up off the bottom breaking the surface to get a breath then squat to drop under the water. Once you are comfortable with bobbing in place with more than just your head emerging, look for your buddy. Let them know that on the next turn, instead of bobbing straight back up, you are going to bob in their direction. When they have been alerted, on the squat, turn toward them and jump toward them. Try not to bump them but wind up standing up next to them.

For fun, the buddies could try to slap a congratulatory high five at the peak of their bobs.

3.3 Prone Float and Recovery

In this activity, the buddies will one at a time practice floating face down and then recover to a standing position. The active buddy brings their arms together over their head, leans forward, takes a breath, and with a little flex of their feet assumes a horizontal position in the pool. The body may glide forward a bit. Arms should be extended out from the body to stop forward movement. The active buddy should relax their body while slowly exhaling their breath. At this point you are floating. After about 5 to 10 seconds, the recovery portion of this exercise begins. It's at this time that the observing/assisting buddy should be nearby and close enough to lend a hand as needed. The arms start the recovery by pushing downward into the water while continuing to exhale. At the same time begin bending you knees, tucking your feet up toward their stomach, and raise your head. When the head is completely emerged, the feet should be extended down to the pool floor and you take a breath. Buddies should practice this until they are comfortable with the recovery portion.

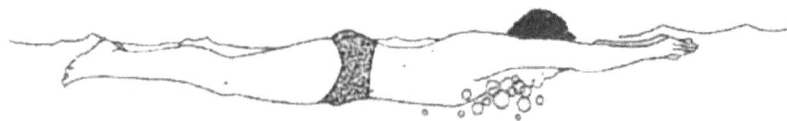

Figure 23 Face or Prone Float

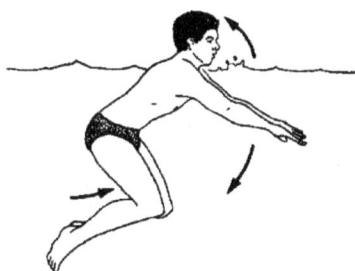

Figure 24 Recovery from a Prone Float

3.4   Back or Supine float

In this activity, women generally have an advantage over men. In shallow water, begin by inhaling a large breath of air. Lean backwards until you become horizontal floating on your back. Do nothing. Relax. If your legs begin to sink, move to shallower water to let them rest on the bottom or place a pull-buoy, kickboard, or noodle under the small of your back positioned to keep your legs afloat.   When you exhale, you will begin to sink so take a quick breath as needed. Relax the muscles of your neck, shoulders, arm. The water's buoyancy will take the weight off as you assume a neutral position slightly bobbing in the water with each breath.

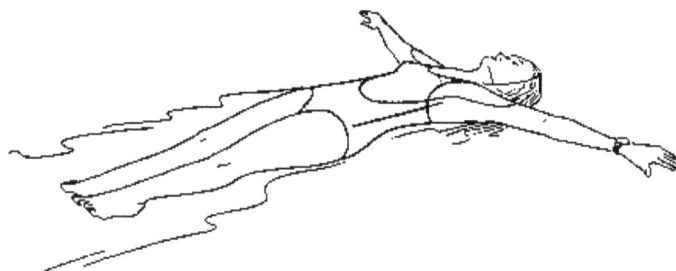

Figure 25 Back float position

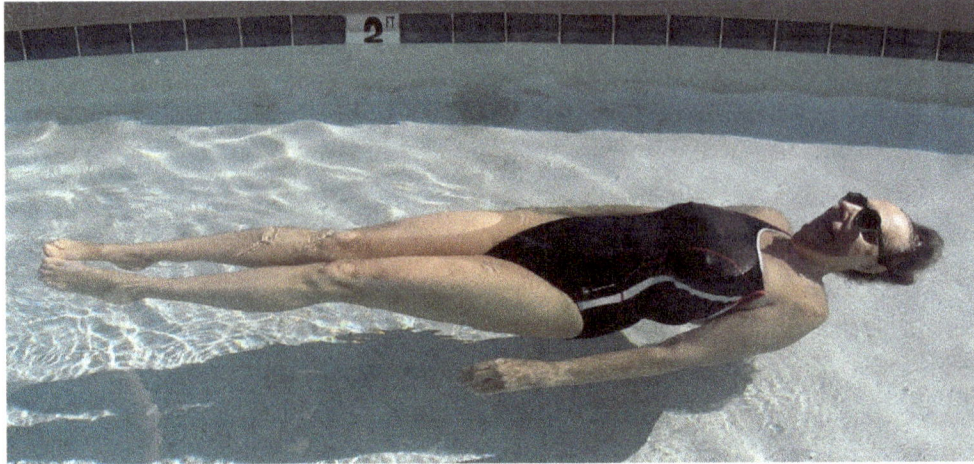

Figure 26 Dr. Jane Katz demonstrating the back float

For recovery, bend forward with your hands sweeping backwards and down. If you are in shallow water, just sit up or stand up after rolling onto your stomach. If you are in deep water, begin an alternating frog kick (eggbeater) to hold yourself up or roll over and begin swimming with a large kick to get started.

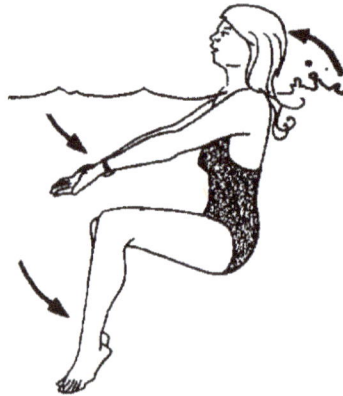

Figure 27 Back float recovery

Your buddy can offer suggestions through observation when you recover a standing position or help right you. Once the buddies are comfortable with the recovery, they can both float at the same time. You keep an eye out for each other.

The fun part of this exercise is getting the rest in an aquatic environment where you can't hear the phone ring or anyone talking to you. If you are outdoors, count the birds flying overhead. If you

3.5   Push-off Glide

In this lesson students learn how to launch themselves properly to begin a swim stroke. The buddies are together in the pool. The active buddy is positioned by the wall and the observe/assist buddy is about 10 feet away in the direction of the glide. The active buddy assumes a position with their arm outstretched over their head. The thumbs are together with the arms touching their ears. The buddy is bent forward at the waist. After inhaling, the knees are flexed to begin a push off with their toes, one foot or two feet can be placed against the pool wall. After further bending forward, the forehead touches the water, the legs are quickly straightened, and the process of exhalation begins. The push-off is completed and the glide has begun. The active buddy is gliding toward the observer/assist buddy. Upon slowing down the active buddy draws the knees forward, pressed downward with the hands to lift the head, and extends the legs to the floor to stand up. The buddies switch positions and the other buddy returns to the wall in the same fashion. Repeat until the buddies are comfortable with this exercise.

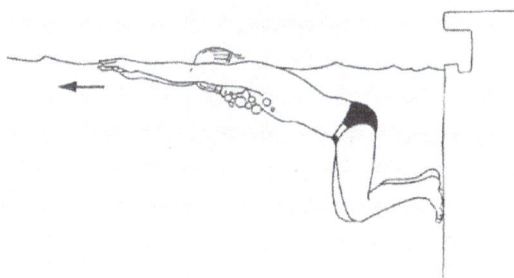

Figure 28 Push Off and Glide

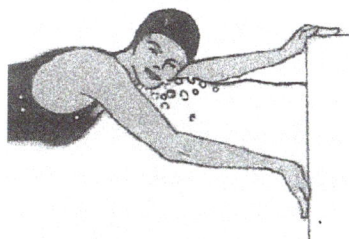

Bracket Position

Figure 29 Prone position wall support

3.6 Flutter Kick

The main source of propulsion for the glide is the push off from the wall. What the flutter kick allows is for the swimmer to move along steadily after the glide slows down. This is a movement done with the feet as indicated by the word "kick". The flutter aspect is obtained by moving your legs in a beating motion up and down. You alternate the leg movement so when one leg is moving up, the other leg is moving down close together. The flutter effect is obtained by the rapid movement of the legs by not kicking the legs more than about 12 inches. The rapid movement is the flutter kick.

While you are kicking the water, you won't be going anywhere if you don't modify the kick slightly. On the downward beat the knee bends slightly and at the end of the stroke the knee and the leg is straight. The swimmer should use a motion somewhat like kicking a ball at the bottom of the downward kick adding a little emphasis to the kick. The knee is straight at this point of the kick. This motion gives downward thrust and power to the kick. On the upward movement of the leg, the foot doesn't change positions and is pointed straight in line with the lower leg. The knee is straight after the end of the downward movement but changes position to bent by the end of the upward kick. The foot does not change positions that much. This adds backward thrust during the upward kick. The foot may break the surface causing splashing which is expected. Toes always remain pointed to maximize the water movement.

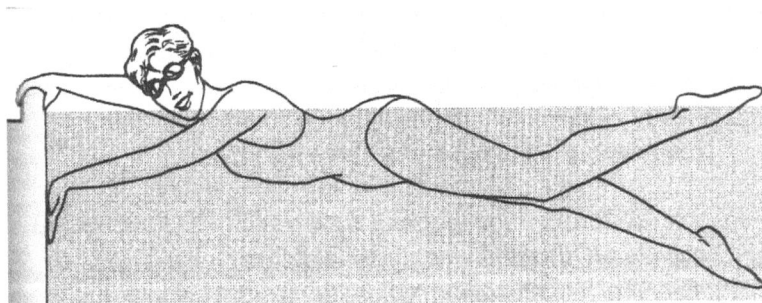

Figure 30 Flutter Kick (left leg poised to begin down beat)

That is the theory. Now for the practice. The active buddy takes the push-off position on the wall while the observing buddy moves about 2 or 3 body lengths away. This is the away location. The active buddy pushes off in a prone glide slowly exhaling. As the glide slows down, the flutter kick should be started to finish the distance or until the air runs out in which case the observing buddy adjusts the away position. Upon reaching the observing buddy, the active buddy rests a moment to catch a breath. Then turns around, squats, and pushes off the bottom to kick back to the wall. This second half of the exercise is more difficult.

For fun the buddies can play a guessing game where the swimmer on the push off picks a number between 1 to 10 and the observing buddy tries to guess it. Without revealing the number, the active buddy upon reaching the wall announces "higher" or "lower", then pushes off again to obtain the observing buddy's new guess when the active buddy reaches the away position. When the observing buddy finally guesses the number, the observing buddy squats, pushes off the bottom to kick to the wall. The game repeats with the buddies in new positions.

3.7   Kickboard Practice

This exercise is similar to the flutter kick exercise. It is used to practice the flutter kick. Here the swimmer holds onto the front portion of a kickboard with both hand while standing next to the pool wall. One leg can be placed on the wall to assist with a push off. The board is placed on the water in front of the swimmer who grasps the board at the round end. When the push off occurs, the active buddy launches forward from the flexing of the knees or pushing off the wall. The kickboard supports the head above the water allowing swimmers to see where they are going and breathe. The laps would be across the shallow end of the pool or width (shorter) distance.

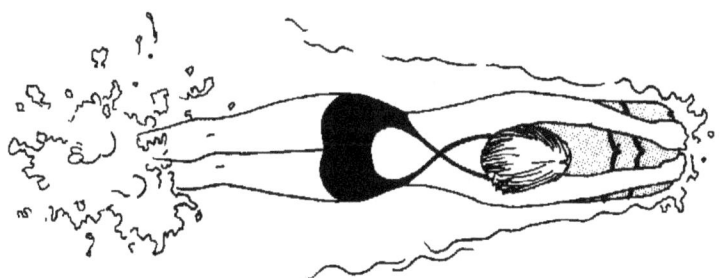

Figure 31 Practicing the flutter kick with a kickboard

The observing buddy can be stationed at the opposite end who awaits the arrival of a kickboard retrieved from the active buddy when the first lap is completed. When this buddy arrives at the original side the exercise is complete. If both buddies have kickboards, the buddy's wait for the arrival of the other before beginning their next lap. The exercise would have a specific number of laps to be completed. Since any kickboard exercise normally supports the head out of the water, conversation is encouraged. Fins can help new swimmers improve their kicking skills when to keep their leg straight and when to bend their knees.

For a fun competition, kickboards of different colors are stacked at either end. The buddies start at opposite ends of the pool pushing a kickboard in the water at the same time in opposite directions, the buddies push the kickboards from one side of the pool to the other, place that kickboard on the pool desk taking the other color kickboard with them on the return trip until the two piles of kickboards are switched. Cheering and encouragement is allowed.

3.8   Sculling techniques

This lesson is about an underwater stroke/skill that provides propulsion, stability, and support. The buddies are in the water together. While standing the active buddy begins by placing their hands on top of the water with the elbows bent so the palms of their hands are facing downward. Push the water away as you rotate your thumbs to pointed down. You only need to move your hands about 6 to 8 inches. You should create a wave radiating away from you with your hands thumbs down as your hands sweep the water. Now with the hands in this extended position, rotate the thumb upward and sweep the water together. The fingers dig into the water here. This is the basic movement: away, together, repeat.

Now, for the next step, immerse your body up to your neck and repeat this motion only include some up and down movement of the hands by adding a circular motion at the end. When the hands move out, at the end as the thumb needs to turn up, plunge the hand down gradually about 3" or 4" as it rotates. On the return sweep, gradually raise the hand toward the surface so when it reaches the point where the thumb should point down, it can again be plunged down into the water. You are drawing a figure 8 with both hands at the same time.

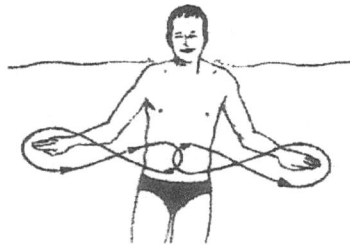

Figure 32 Sculling

Our next step is to launch you using just your hands for support. If you are in shallow water, you could be sitting or kneeling and in deeper water standing. Lean back allowing the angle at the elbows to increase so your hands stay underwater keeping the palms of your hand parallel to the water surface (the angle of the bend at the wrist also increases). Lift your feet off the bottom as you lean back. If you start sinking, increase the tempo of the sweep. If you are pushing down at the ends of the rotation, you will support yourself…observing/assisting buddy, pay attention here. Your hands should be cycling through their stroke about even with your wrist when your feet break the water. Your body is straight, and the angle of the wrist is also straight.

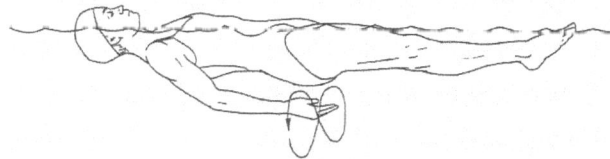

Figure 33 Sculling (both hands) while floating.

Now you can experiment with movement by subtle changes in the angle of wrist bend. To go forward bend the wrist down slightly. To go backward, bend the wrist up slightly. To rotate in a circle, have the wrists bend in opposite direction all the time sculling the water. The goal once the buddies become comfortable with this is to be able to move forward, back and rotate in place.

For fun the entire class can play the Ancient World Maritime War game. The main rule is if one buddy T-bones another, the struck buddy is sunk and out of the game.

Chapter 4 The *Alternating* Strokes

4.1 Introduction

Swim strokes can be divided into two types of motion: *alternating and simultaneous.*

The crawl stroke is an alternating stroke: As you glide your left arm forward to catch the water, your right arm is at the end of the pull phase. And while you bring your left arm through the pull, your right arm is recovering above the water. Similarly, your left leg is at the highest portion of the kick motion, while your right leg is at its deepest position. When you swim backstroke, the same alternating motion applies: As your leg hand enters the water, your right hand is at your hip, leaving the water. Your legs also kick alternately to each other.

4.2 The Crawl Stroke

The crawl stroke uses everything you have learn up to this point: your breathing, the prone float, and the flutter kick. This is a stroke seen in the Olympics, the beach, and at local pools. It is the fastest stoke known to mankind. It is called the crawl stroke because it looks like you are crawling through the water. The backstroke is the crawl stroke when swimming on your back (supine position). There are differences in the breathing and arm motions, but both use alternating arm and kick strokes.,

4.2.1 The Crawl Stroke Arm Movements.

This stroke uses a rotation of your arms through the water, alternating positions where one arm is in front of you, plunged underwater and the other arm is alongside your waist about to be lifted above the water to return to the front. This rotation of the arms is much like the kick where one leg is up about to stroke down through the water and the other leg is down about to kick up to the surface. Because the kick is shorter, for every arm stroke you use about two kicks. The arm stroke has three major aspects: the CATCH, PULL, and the RECOVERY. The power for the stroke comes from your shoulder rotation accommodating the movement of your arm through the water and your breathing. If you are a veteran, you will be used to saluting. In the recovery portion of the arm stroke the hand passes by your face as if you were executing a salute. Veterans have been practicing this swim stroke for years.

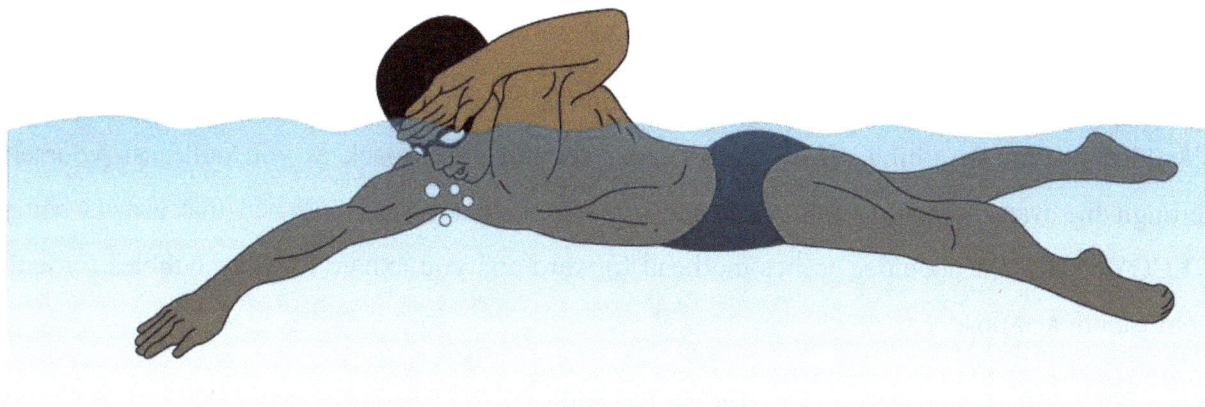

Figure 34 The crawl stroke

4.2.2   Breathing Technique

Swim instructors and lifeguards often hear people say, "I can swim but I just can't breathe." Breathing while swimming the crawl stroke involves a technic called rhythmic breathing. It is the secret to swimming more than one lap before stopping at the wall to catch your breath. We have practiced this technique on land and in the water: while your face is in the water, turn your head to one side, right or left, which ever is comfortable for you to inhale; then turning your face back into the water to exhale. While swimming, the head turn (to inhale) is done in rhythm with the arm stroke PULL.

As the arm pulls underwater past your face, turn your head as if to watch the arm move down to your waist. Getting your mouth just above the water is when you inhale a gulp of air. Your head when turned helps to push the water aside allowing you to open your mouth. You can see this effect by forming your hand into a shallow cup then swishing your hand through the water with the back of the hand leading the swish: the water level behind the hand is lower that the water around it. If you swallow water, stop, stand up and cough it out then try again after pushing off from the bottom to pick up some momentum.

When the arm reaches the waist, the RECOVERY portion begins. This is when you exhale. How long should you exhale? Slowly enough to last until your next breath but not so fast that your become starved for oxygen or you begin turning your head to breath on both sides. If you are well oxygenated, you can hold your breath until the arms rotate enough to accommodate your inhaling.

You hold your breath when pushing off underwater so a short period of time can be allowed while swimming.

Another way to time your breathing: while swimming, keep your head in synch with which ever shoulder you are breathing off of. When your shoulder goes back as you pull/push yourself through the water, the head follows it and you catch your breath. When that arm is being RECOVERED, the shoulder pushes the head forward and you exhale forming bubbles through your mouth and nose.

Were you to lift your head up, you lose the swishing effect of the arm stroke and it changes the position of your body in the water. The more in line with the surface of the water, the less resistance your body creates as you move through the water. Lifting your head drops your feet lower creating even more drag slowing your progress through the water.

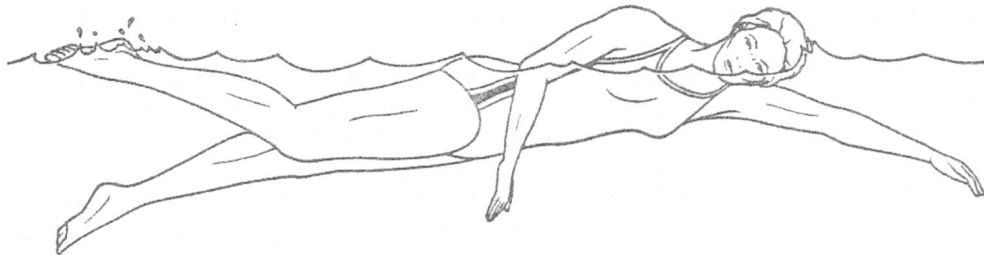

Figure 35 Swimmer inhaling during the PULL portion of the arm stroke

4.2.3   More arm stroke techniques

The whole body including your breathing affect the arm stroke, this section concerns details about how the arm stroke has been modified to emphasis the whole-body swimming effect.

The PULL starts with the CATCH of the water by the hands. Your hand may enter the water straight to lessen resistance but just like when you practiced sculling, you catch more water when the hands are slightly cupped by turning your thumbs up. Your hand shape will change as you stroke through the water. You catch the water deep in front of you along an extended centerline of the body. Your body may rotate led by the shoulders, but the body does not bend. Just like a bicycle is stiff so that the external parts can apply the force they are developing to pull your body along, keeping the body straight and in-line minimizes resistance.

You scoop the water allowing the hand to gradually turn back toward your face as if you were going to drink the water, arm slightly crocked as you are turning onto your side at this point in the water. When the hand turns and the forearm is at 90 degrees to the body, the hand and the forearm form a larger cup swishing the water out and away from your chest. Then with the arm still cocked at 90 degrees, the hand flattens, and the arm becomes a paddle to swept directly behind you. Your hip has by the time rotated up as the other hand has entered the water for a deep plunge. Your upper arm exercises the biceps muscles as you draw the water toward your body then the triceps take over for the PULL completion. The pattern the hand follows is an "S" curve. With the shoulder rotation, the whole-body movement is very much like a baseball player's swing at a pitched ball. Where the hand entered the water measured to where the hand leaves the water is about the length of your hand. Your hand and arm are like a propeller blade's twist that corkscrews thru the air. You are using the lift created as your arm pulls through the water as if you were crawling up steps made of the water's resistance.

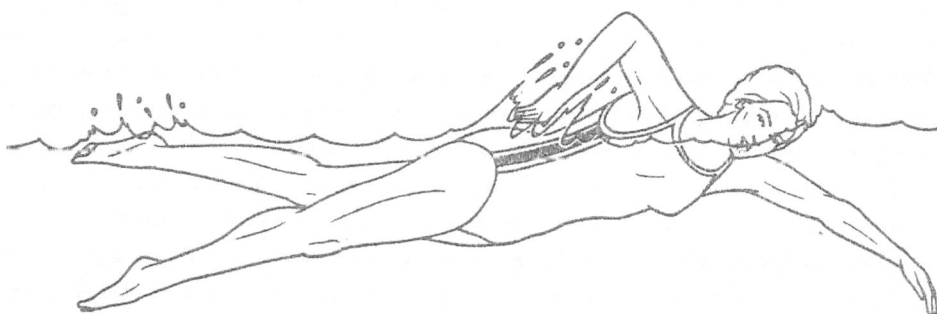

Figure 36 left arm: CATCH/PULL, right arm: RECOVERY, ROTATION inhaling

The RECOVER is with the elbow high giving you a weight more effectively counter-balancing your rotation like an ice skater controls the speed of their rotations with the positions of their arms. The hand enters the water like a stiletto not far from your face and slightly ahead of the eyes. You could say it's a salute in honor to your next stroke. As the forearm and upper arm enter the water, they twist the thumbs down. Some splashing it to be incurred as the arm begins to bend to cup the water.

4.2.4   Shoulder rotation

Shoulder rotation is key to putting power into your arm stroke. As you rotate your arms through the water, allows your shoulders to follow the motion your body you create by plunging one arm forward deep into the water for the catch of the PULL. You could even exaggerate the motion which causes the other shoulder to lift-up easier as you exhale. If your shoulders have little rotation, you will find your recover stroke may drag through the water with a poor arm entry. Poor shoulder rotation may cause shoulder injuries over time where it becomes painful to reach above your head. Make your crawl arm stroke less stressful by rotating the shoulder so you don't push your arms into the plane of the back.

A good shoulder rotation helps the hips rotate increasing the power of your kicks. The hips rotate in synch with the shoulders changing from a strictly vertical up and down kick. Your kick will have a longer travel keeping the kick shallower creating less drag.

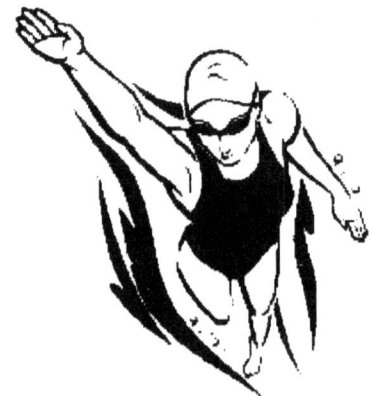

Figure 37 Swimmer is thrusting the hand forward to catch the water and is about to rotate her body.

4.2.5   Tips for the Crawl Stroke

1. CATCH: a streamlined hand water-entry doesn't splash
2. RECOVERY: keep elbows high
3. PULL: extend the arm all the way to your waist
4. RHYTHMIC BREATHING: turn head to one side only
5. KICK: move legs in rhythm with your stroke
6. BODY MOVEMENT: rotate all the way down to your toes
7. START: push off with a glide to a prone float to begin your stroke

4.3   The Back Stroke

Imagine you were about to swim a lap and after you pushed off, you popped up to the surface on your back. The only stroke you knew was the crawl stroke. You then began swimming the crawl stroke upside-down, alternating the arm stokes, rotating your shoulders, and kicking as usual and finding it way easier to get a breath. That is the back stroke and with a slight modification to the PULL and RECOVERY movements, it's the favorite go-to stroke for many a swimmer. You may find you like a nose clip to keep water from entering your nose when you inhale.

In the backstroke, your back is arched to keep your hair submerged with the face looking up, enough so that you can peek forward just a bit to find the backstroke flags about 5 yards from the end of the pool. You also are watching the lane lines to keep in the middle of the lane. Don't take more than 3 strokes further past the backstroke flags. Throw one final arm forward to glide into the wall. Modern rules allow back strokers to rotate over onto their stomach at this time.

The arm stroke for the backstroke. In the PULL, your arms enter the water with the hand and fingers pointed down as much as possible while the swimmer shoulders leans into this thrust pushing the arm at least one foot under the water. With the arm bent at 90 degrees, the hand is rotated up toward the surface and away from the body, much like the crawl stroke swish as if you were throwing a ball to your feet, The thumbs during the PULL which were pointed down are rotate up during this swish and as they past the waist they are rotated down again. Finally, the arm is struck hard to the waist in the final push because your body has rotated to allow the other arm to enter the water. For the RECOVERY, bring your hand up the centerline of your body sliding outward high over the head preparing to plunge the arm with the hand bend backward into the water. The alternating kick is with toes pointed as much as possible not breaking the surface.

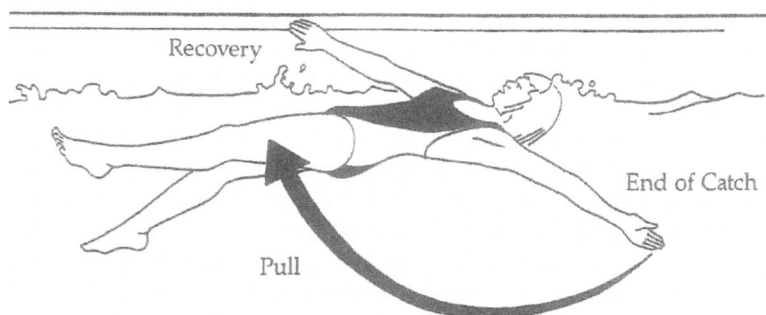

Figure 38 Modern backstroke

Chapter 5 Symmetrical Strokes

5.1 Introduction

The breaststroke is a simultaneous stroke. The motion of each arm mirrors the other, moving symmetrically at the midline of your body. Likewise, the motion of your legs mirrors each other. In the breaststroke, your arms trace a heart-shaped motion, beginning above your head and then under your chest, pulling you forward. Your legs mimic a frog kick, simultaneously apart and then snapping together, pushing you forward. When the motions of your arms and legs are timed correctly, you move smoothly and efficiently through the water exhaling underwater in a prone float position.

The butterfly, the most dramatic stroke, also has simultaneous movement. Both hands enter the water in front of your head, pull through the water in an "S" shaped pull under your body, and exit the water at your hips. Your feet stay together, pushing the water backwards as you kick, propelling you forward.

The breaststroke, one of the oldest strokes, and the butterfly stroke, one of the newest competitive strokes known to mankind, are performed in a prone position using symmetrical kicks and arm strokes. Breathing becomes somewhat easier by lifting your head straight up out of the water. The leg strokes differ from each other with one thrusting the legs backwards and the other moving the legs up and down smoothly like the tail fins of a dolphin and a porpoise.

5.2   The Breaststroke

In chapter two, Aquatic Fitness, you were introduced to an exercise called "Leg Lifts". This was an exercise to strength your abdominal muscles. To learn the leg stroke for the breaststroke, assume the position for "Leg Lifts" along the pool wall only turn over on your stomach (prone position). You can onto the pool with two hands or use the bracket position to support yourself. The RECOVERY portion on the breaststroke is the same: pull your legs up together as though you were squatting. The STROKE begins by turning your feet at a 90-degree angle from each other holding the heels together as well as the knees (for streamlining). The STROKE finishes with quick extension of the legs in a slight semicircle until they meet when the legs are fully extended. As the STROKE occurs, the feet twist slightly to allow the broadest portion of the foot to scoop as much water as possible. This kick is known as the "Whip kick,"

5.3   The Breaststroke Mechanics and Timing the Arm Stroke

The plane of the hips and legs at their furthest extension with toes pointed like a ballerina, form a platform for the arm stroke action to push the upper body up out of the water. The arm stroke begins at the moment the breaststroke leg STROKE begins. The arms are fully extended and hand cupped together at the beginning of the arm stroke. As the kick occurs, the hands break apart, turning thumbs down, each arm sweeping out and down until they approach a 90-degree angle at the elbow. At this point, the hands push down and are drawn together at your chest support the lifting of the head above the water. With your head at this highest point above the water is when the breaststroker has a chance to inhale. The hands are in a position as if you might be saying a prayer. This is a description of the arm stroke PULL combined with the head movement for the breaststroke. The RECOVERY begins with the arms lifting up somewhat as if to dive back into the water. The head points down to follow the hands until they are fully extended. During the arm stroke recovery, the legs are also being recovered. There is a continuous forward movement of the body. There is no rotation but there is a motion that has the swimmer's body rocking up and down through the water that is similar to a butterfly dolphin kick.

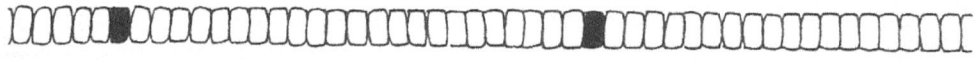

1.

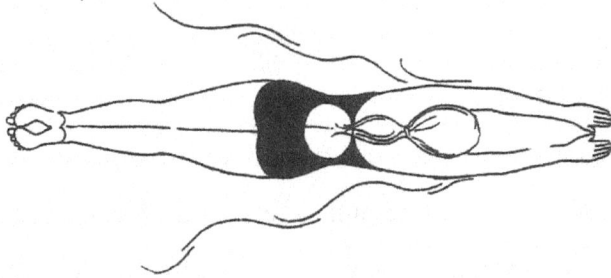

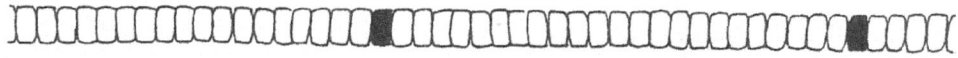

2.

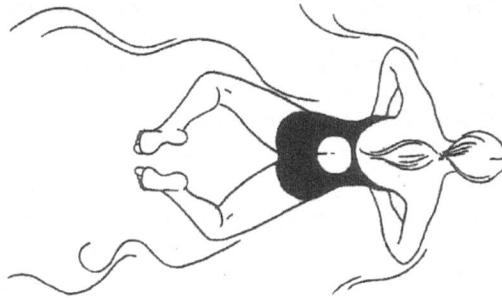

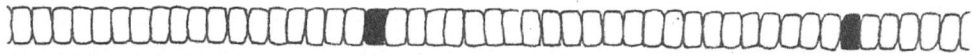

3.

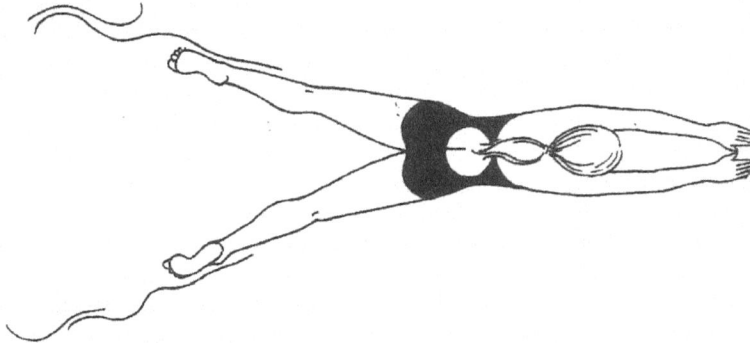

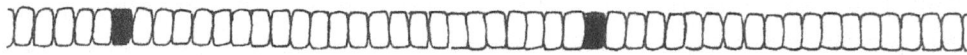

4.

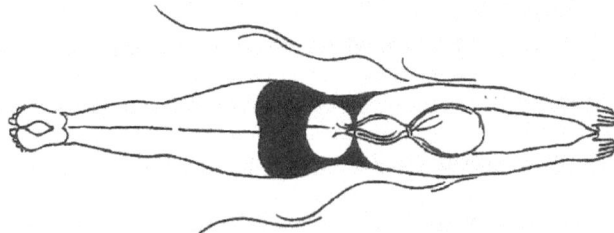

Figure 39 Breaststroke sequence

5.4   The Butterfly Stroke: Swimming Like A Dolphin

In this exercise swimmers practice a basic skill of butterfly swimming: arm recovery.   The swimmer begins by squatting in shallow water then pushes off the bottom, jumping up and forward with their arms by their side as they emerge from the water.   Before their head reenters the water several feet forward, the arms are brought forward to part the water for their head and body to follow.   Underwater, the arms break the dive by corrects the entry to glide forward underwater to set up for the next leap.   The exercise is broken up into parts: learning how to do just one jump/dive then piecing together several once after another.   The arm mechanics are like jumping rope with the rope starting behind your feet and being cast overhead before being pulled under the person's feet in a small jump step.

Here are the essentials: The butterfly arm stroke recovery starts with both hand behind you about a half foot away from your hips.   The arms are thrown up out of the water still away from your body and swish across the water while your head is bent upward to inhale a breath.   The arms point down and toward a point ahead of you that is about 4 inches underwater.   The hands eventually reach the starting position for the PULL portion of the Butterfly stroke forward of your head.

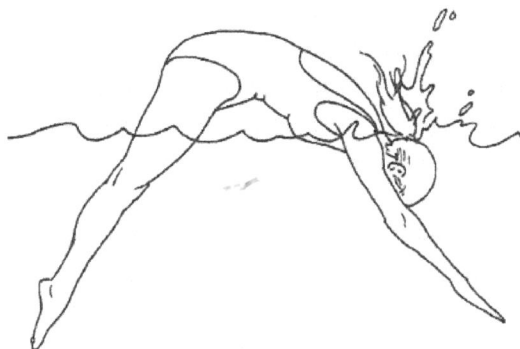

Figure 40 Dolphin dive

5.5   The Dolphin Kick

This kick is a very efficient leg kick used with the butterfly stroke and solo when swimming underwater.   We will discuss the solo underwater dolphin kick used for wall push off or just swimming underwater.   Imagine a small wave that your body follows while floating on the water face down. As the wave travels from your hands (positioned in the prone float over your head) along to your head lifting these body parts up then setting them back down with a slight dip followed by the shoulders, chest, waist, legs and finally your feet. When you do a dolphin kick, your body undulated in the same manner only you are underwater.

You start the dolphin after pushing off underwater with your hands and let the rest of your body swings in rhythm as you mimic this wave only when the wave gets to your feet, accentuated the leg movement, so you can kick downward with power. There is some bending at the waist as you flex along. To resurface, the hands stroke together, swing out wide then whip down to your sides almost meeting under your stomach causing the head to emerge as you arch your back upward. There are usually two kicks to every arm stroke. A small dolphin kick as you execute the PULL of the arm stroke, then a large kick to help you lift your arms and head about the water to breath and execute the RECOVERY portion of the arm stroke.

Chapter 6 PTSD

W.E.T.s 4 VETS® is a program to benefit local communities. What makes this aquatic program special is that it brings together veterans and civilians that has a therapeutic effect on the mind, body, and spirit of the participants. What is post-traumatic stress disorder (PTSD)? It is a serious potentially debilitating condition that can occur in people who have experienced or witnessed a natural disaster, serious accident, terrorist incident, the sudden death of a loved one, war, and violent personal assault such as rape or other life-threatening events[1]. This is the "what happened" that is the source of the syndrome.

The Department for Veteran Affairs estimates the number of veterans with PTSD by service era: Desert Storm was 12% while the Vietnam War was 15%[2]. Over 600,000 veterans have received treatment for PTSD thru March of 2014. This is double the total number in 2006[3]. This is an increasing phenomenon. Approximately 20 percent of Iraqi and Afghanistan veterans have PTSD and depression[4]. This is a significant problem.

In meeting and working with veterans it's as important to know the signs of PTSD symptoms as it is to know how to rescue a swimmer from drowning. Here is a condensed list[5]:

- Feeling:
  - upset by things that remind you of what happened
  - emotionally cut off from others, losing interest in things you used to care about
  - constantly on guard, irritated or having angry outbursts
- Having
  - difficulty sleeping
  - Having trouble concentrating
  - nightmares, vivid memories, or flashbacks of the event
- Being jumpy or easily startled
- Or feeling like it's happening all over again

[1] Anxiety and Depression Association of America, www.adaa.org.
[2] Veterans and PTSD, http://www.veteransandptsd.com/PTSD-statistics.html.
[3] Claire Ansberry, *Veterans seek health benefits from PTSD decades after War, WSJ, Nov. 28, 2014.*
[4] Rand Corporation, http://www.rand.org/pubs/monographs/2008/RAND_MG720.pdf.
[5] "*MakeTheConnection.net* is an online resource designed to connect Veterans, their family members and friends, and other supporters with information, resources, and solutions to issues affecting their lives." Veterans Crisis Line 800-273-8255. Website: https://maketheconnection.net.

6.1   Treatment

Everyone reacts to traumatic events differently. Each person is unique in his or her ability to manage fear and stress and to cope with the threat posed by a traumatic event or situation. You don't have to be a veteran to have symptoms like PTSD. First, you must be diagnosed by a doctor. There are no lab tests for PTSD so once physical illness reasons are ruled out, individuals are referred to a psychiatrist, psychologist, or other mental health professional who rule out other source of psychiatric conditions. The doctor then determines if the symptoms and degree of dysfunction rise to the level of PSTD. Treatment may involve psychotherapy (counseling), medication or both. Medication are antidepressant medication to treat PTSD and control the feelings of anxiety and its associated symptoms[6].

6.2   A personal experience of PTSD:

I served in the U.S. Army Infantry for nearly 5 years. I joined in 2009 and was medically separated after sustaining injuries in combat. Though separating from the military was one of the hardest decisions to make, it was the beginning of a long road to recovery. Among the physical injuries, I was diagnosed with PTSD and TBI. This all made the long transition from the military to a civilian that much more difficult when I returned home. As many veterans' state, when they return the transitional period is the toughest.

When I returned home at the end of 2013, I realized that this transition is going to be hard. I had heard the stories prior to leaving but I didn't have any idea how difficult it could be. One of the biggest hardships was learning how the civilian life works and being part of society. I quickly learned that I was isolating myself from the surrounding and was highly vigilant with the surrounding world This was difficult because it prevented me from taking mass transportation and going into crowded places. I saw myself going weeks without food in my refrigerator because the supermarkets were too crowded to enter. This is when I realized that I had some issues to deal with, but I felt no one will understand. I reached out to some friends and most of them told me they were dealing with the same issues and that was the first sense of peace I had since leaving the military. It was at this point I knew I had to do more to help myself.

After months of physical therapy and mental health therapy, I began to feel slightly at ease. In my mind, I thought this is finally coming to an end. But it wasn't. In fact, I shortly was reminded that this will be an everlasting battle that veterans will endure. I had to step up to do something to help my brothers and sisters returning from service. I began counseling and veteran's advocacy. I was responsible for helping process veterans through the counseling process and linking them to the appropriate services. This gave me a great sense of fulfillment because I was helping the veterans who fell into a huge gray area.

[6] WebMD, Posttraumatic Stress Disorder, website: https://www.webmd.com/mental-health/post-traumatic-stress-disorder#3-6

6.3 W.E.T.s 4 VETS®

Here we will examine what makes W.E.T.s 4 VETS® different and special from other approaches to PTSD. For one, the sessions don't talk about this problem. A second perhaps noticeable difference is it's not just your family and friends taking the class. There are people, civilians taking the course you don't know, at least at the beginning of the session. We don't even talk about acclimating to civilian life but that results happens. You don't forget your service to your country but you're happy to have learned new aquatic skills and look forward to another fun session.

Beyond learning the aquatic skills, you've helped another person acquire these skills just by being there and participating. You learn the skills when you are the active buddy and you then observe and assist the other buddy do likewise. Or it's the other way around, you observe the mistakes or success of your buddy, you help fix or learn from their attempt, and you are the more able to attempt the skill knowing this information. Even in the observing, once you have experienced the skills you've become more knowledgeable about how to do it. It's all new. You get to share this with the most obvious person, the buddy you're partnered with. This is very much like another military saying, "See one, do one, teach one".

You know you are becoming a different person. With just a few sessions you are becoming more confident and eager to take the next step. You are not a leader yet, but you know you are on the right path. You will know how to swim safely, and you will know how to help someone struggling in the water because you've been there.

You've been given goals and you've accomplished them as a team. There is strength in numbers. You are a force multiplier. You not been given complicated tasks but by focusing on the instructions you are able to concentrate on what is important. Your mind is clear. You've learned from the progress in the session that it's important to put first things first else you'll flounder. It's why the class didn't start the first day in the deep end. The question, "How do I get from here to where I want to go" begins with baby steps that upon knowing allows better questions to be asked. You've allowed yourself to learn, which is a great lesson in itself. When you can see your progress, you have become able to judge if it's taking you to where you want to go. These are life lessons. You've taken steps to become a leader.

6.4   Benefits of W.E.T.s 4 VETS®:

Lifetime fitness training	Focus/Concentration/Goas
Acclimate to civilian life	Buoyancy—you weigh less
Snacks/parties/celebrations	Water volleyball and other aquatic games
Meet new friends	Confidence
Rehabilitation	Water's timelessness
Water skills	Drown proofing
Resistance training	Lifetime safety skills

There is no blame or guilt for an individual to feel for having or seeking treatment for PTSD. Some take a route of self-treatment using alcohol. It will work for a while then you'll find yourself servant to two masters, drink and PTSD. Just checking it out is your first step in recovery. You can relieve yourself of inestimable gloom and gain the admiration of your friends and family. There is no loss for individuals if they earnestly seek that healthful and rewarding life they deserve. Go for it.

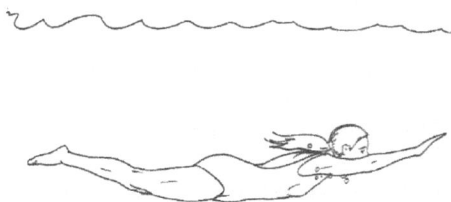

Figure 41 Feeling like Superman…free from gravity and fears

6.5   Summary

A real summary could simply be a list of tasks that the participants in this W.E.T.s 4 VETS® program would have checked off. Did you learn this? Did you learn that and have most of them checked off? In classes, a summary would be a final test.

Those aren't the goals in W.E.T.s 4 VETS®. It runs deeper. We could ask if you had fun? A fair question would be: Did you learn something about aquatic fitness? The real goals for this program run much deeper and our learning knowledge base is certainly useful for drown proofing. You could go on to be a lifeguard, swim instructor, pool manager, aquatic director but these are not the true goals of this program.

It's more how you feel about yourself as compared with the self you were before beginning W.E.T.s 4 VETS®. Everyone is going to feel different about themselves whether they took W.E.T.s 4 VETS® or not simply because they are older, had more experiences, life happened. But in your case, the authors of this manual are hoping that your self has become more aware of relationships, patience, listening, trial and error, recovery, success, or on becoming a better water volleyball player. We're looking for the memories that will stay with you as you move on and traits that can help you build on your character.

We are especially keen on the trial and error and recovery. No one is going to have an error free life, so the question becomes more about your recovery. Here in W.E.T.s 4 VETS®, it's simply about standing up and not drowning. Life will throw more complications at you and it's important to recognize when you are in trouble and to see/find/discover/realize a path to recovery which would be a better you because of it. How do you hold your head up and get that next breath?

This is our summary: Stroke on and take your next breath.

Chapter 7 General Nutrition Recommendations:

The United States Department of Agriculture, (USDA) produces a publication called *Dietary Guidelines for Americans*. The USDA revises this resource every five years.

Key recommendations in the Dietary Guidelines suggest observing a *healthy eating pattern* that accounts for all foods and beverages within an appropriate calorie level.

A *healthy eating pattern* includes:

1. A variety of vegetables from all of the subgroups—dark green, red and orange, legumes (beans and peas), starchy, and other
2. Fruits, especially whole fruits
3. Grains, at least half of which are whole grains
4. Fat-free or low-fat dairy, including milk, yogurt, cheese, and/or fortified soy beverages
5. A variety of protein foods, including seafood, lean meats and poultry, eggs, legumes (beans and peas), and nuts, seeds, and soy products
6. Oils

A *healthy eating pattern* limits: Saturated fats and trans fats, added sugars, and sodium. To help implement these guidelines, the USDA has created a resource called MyPlate:

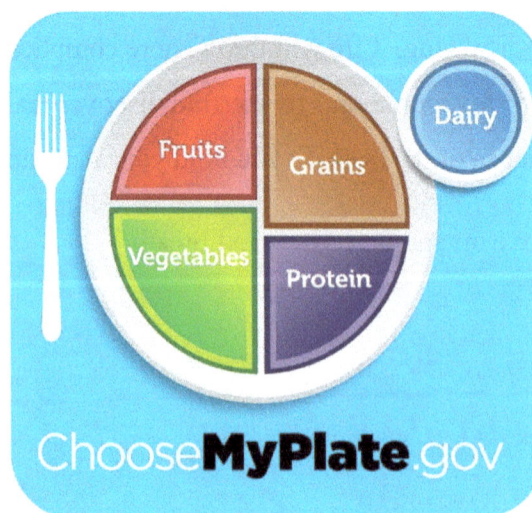

MyPlate visually displays what a healthy plate of food should look like. Notice that vegetables and fruits fill half the plate. While focusing on variety, it is also recommended that you include different colors of foods, especially vegetables and fruits.

What about eating before a WETs4VETS workout?

You should eat something before your workout, so that you don't get hungry before you are out of the pool and dressed. Eating two to three hours before a workout is ideal. If you need to eat just before you go to the pool, eat foods that are light and sit well in your stomach. Carbohydrate foods give your energy, protein helps maintain your energy. Therefore, try to eat a combination of foods containing carbohydrates and protein. A high fat or heavy meal, prior to your pool workout, may make you feel bloated or uncomfortably full in the water.

What about drinking water?

Bring a Water Bottle with you, to your WETs4VETS session. By keeping a water bottle close by (on the pool deck), you'll be able to hydrate when needed. Be sure that your water bottle is not breakable (many facilities do not allow glass bottles). Carbonated beverages (sodas) are not recommended. What is recommended for hydration prior and during sports activities vary, depend on the individual person, the intensity of the activity, temperature and humidity. A general recommendation is to drink about two cups of water 2 - 3 hours prior to the activity. Try to drink water throughout your workout, before you feel thirsty.

Are Sports Drinks Recommended?

WETs4VETS sessions are most likely to be of low or moderate activity. Hydrating with water is sufficient for most participants. Intense workouts, or activities in high temperature and/or high humidity require higher and more frequent fluid intake. Sports beverages may be recommended to replace electrolytes and energy, in addition to fluid.

Online resources include:

https://www.dietaryguidelines.gov/
https://www.choosemyplate.gov/
https://www.myhealth.va.gov/mhv-portal-web/eat-wisely
https://www.nutrition.va.gov/
https://www.move.va.gov/

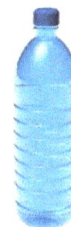

Chapter 8 Miscellaneous

8.1 Testimonials from veteran students

Dr. Katz's W.E.T.'s 4 VETS® program has been invaluable to me. As I and many others can attest getting in the pool makes coming home from war easier for our military service members, veterans, and their families. The unique program that Dr. Katz has designed has given us increased confidence, family, and social connections and to some, learning how to live with a new physical adaption. It has improved mental health for some of our veterans, and a few have shared with me even recovery from addiction. I would like to personally thank Dr. Jane Katz for her whole-hearted support of all her W.E.T.'s 4 VETS® activities that have benefited our John Jay student veterans so much.

This program is truly inspiring and a great help to student veterans. The more people that are made aware of this program, the better. There are many people at John Jay College and the rest of CUNY Schools who could benefit from this terrific program. I've tried to take a leading role representing the John Jay College community as a support to help connect the civilian students with our veteran students. John Jay College is a huge military supporter, and I realized there was a compelling need to help veterans returning from Iraq and Afghanistan...I believe Dr. Katz's program that she has implemented to create a holistic mind, body, and spiritual wellness to the John Jay veteran population is like no other. She has such a dedication to our veteran population and has had a huge impact on them. She helps our student veterans prepare for a purposeful life after the military! Dr. Katz I salute you and your great program W.E.T.'s 4 VETS® and all that you do! Kudos and continue your unflagging devotion to our VETERANS. They need you!!!

The W.E.T.'s 4 VETS® program is an essential program that has helped me with physical injuries that I personally have. The program has helped me emotionally as well. It's as if when I get in the water all my pent-up stress and worries evaporate. The setting to talk to others while working out creates a happy, jolly atmosphere which helps me to relax and enjoy the moments in life. Dr. Katz is an exceptional person. Her presence and joy to serve others shows in how much she cares for us as individuals as she joins in the workout sessions herself. I hope the program can grow and get additional funding to support it as it will certainly help other Vets in need of therapy and be a great asset to connect and have people to talk to and discuss what we're feeling on a day to day basis.

I discovered Dr. Jane Katz W.E.T.s 4 VETS® program where she uses water activities in a therapeutic manner. Her program not only gave me a safe space amongst other students and veterans, but it helps me in my recovery process mentally and physically. I had sustained a severe back injury that had left me paralyzed from the waist down on my left side. I was only recently cleared for water therapy. So, when I found her program, I knew then that I would be very involved because I had multiple purposes. I shared my story to my battle buddies. I get the much-needed physical therapy from the water activities. This program was my god send! It gives me the sense of purpose I needed.

8.2   Press Coverage

The New York Times

City Room
Blogging From the Five Boroughs

Sweat | Making the Water a Comfort Zone

BY COREY KILGANNON   JULY 31, 2010 7:30 AM

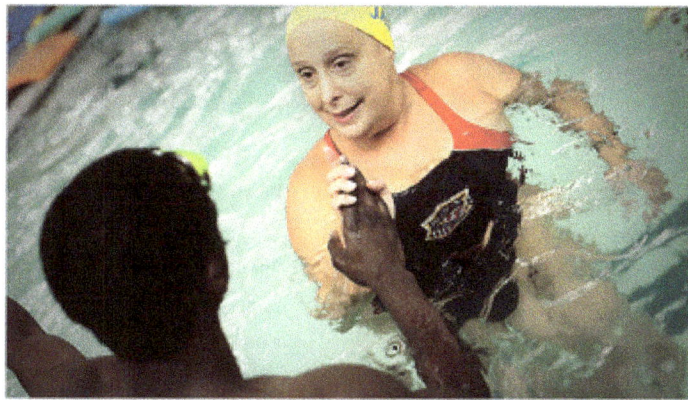

Keith Bedford for The New York Times **AFLOAT** Jane Katz, who has taught swimming in the City University system for 46 years, instructing teenage inmates at John Jay College.

"I AM NOT going in there," said the trembling teenage girl standing at the shallow end of the pool. With her were a half-dozen other girls equally embarrassed to be paraded out in bathing suits and threatened with a swimming lesson.

Work it Out
Sweat is a new biweekly series about sports. Post a Comment »

Down in the water was a hopelessly cheery woman, more than 50 years their senior, flipping around as fluidly as a porpoise. She was Jane Katz, 67, who has been teaching New Yorkers how to swim since the bobby socks era. Ignoring the protestations of the group, who were inmates incarcerated under the city's juvenile justice system, she urged them into the pool at the John Jay College of Criminal Justice in Manhattan.

The teenagers, from the Marolla Group Home, a correctional center in the Bronx, were part of a swimming program that Dr. Katz helped set up 16 years ago for boys and girls in detention. She volunteers her time and pays several lifeguards to help, mostly from her own pocket.

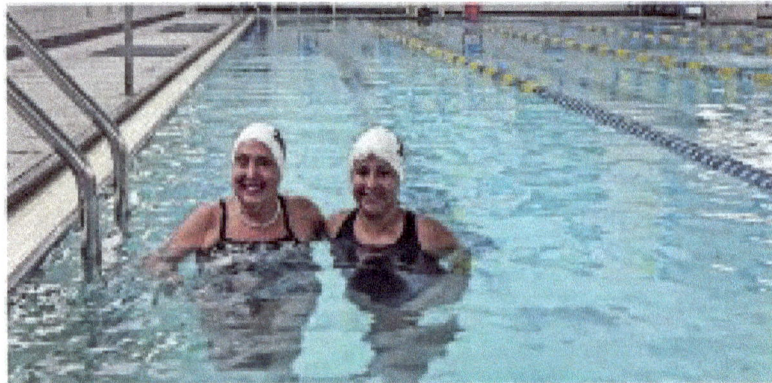

Asphalt Green swimmer Jane Katz (left) started W.E.T.s 4 VETS at John Jay College in New York City in 2012. She estimates her classes have helped nearly a thousand student-veterans, including Cinttia Moreno (right), learn to swim or become better swimmers.
Sarah Morgano

Army veteran Jonathan Martinez, 27, likes how the classes feel on his injured body. He fractured several vertebrae in a fall during his deployment to the eastern border of Pakistan, where he helped stop traffic flow among different factions of the Taliban. When he left the Army in 2013, he enrolled at John Jay and joined Katz's class. He's never stopped going. "I enjoy the physical activity, and I love how comfortable I feel with Jane," he says. "She gives me a place to shine like I'm the best swimmer in the world." Before W.E.T.s 4 VETS here, Martinez only knew how to keep his head above water. "Now I've doubled my speed in freestyle, and I've started learning the other strokes," he says.

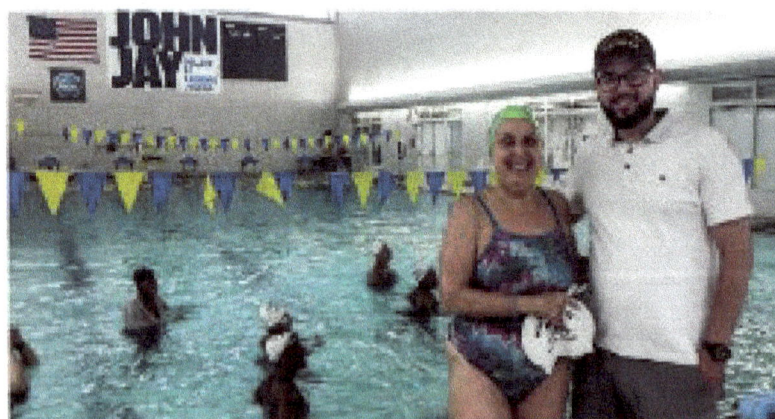

Jonathan Martinez served four years in the Army and suffered injuries to his spine during his deployment to Afghanistan in 2013. He has since learned how to swim through W.E.T.s 4 VETS at John Jay College.
Courtesy of Jonathan Martinez

Courtesy Swimmer Magazine, *Salute to Swimming*, September-October 2017.

The New York Times

FIT CITY

Immersion Therapy at the Pool, for Vets and Civilians

By Lindsay Crouse   July 13, 2017

Splashing in an indoor swimming pool in Manhattan, a group of young men and women tried to keep their heads under water for more than a few moments before they came back up for air. Some of them had already acquired the skills to shoot down rockets and operate tanks while serving as American soldiers in the Middle East. Now they were learning to swim.

Hopping into the pool to join them, an exuberant septuagenarian in a blue swimsuit bellowed orders at her charges, a mix of veterans and students at John Jay College of Criminal Justice. Some were learning to swim for the first time, while others were there to perfect their techniques or for therapeutic or rehabilitative reasons.

"Who are we?" she asked.

"WETs 4 Vets," the swimmers replied in unison, military style, as they treaded water in an ever-expanding circle. Then they started chanting "John Jay" in syncopated staccato, laughing as they grew more comfortable in the water. American flags protruded from their caps like feathers from a fedora. (WET stands for water exercise techniques.)

8.1   Milestones for Women Inclusion

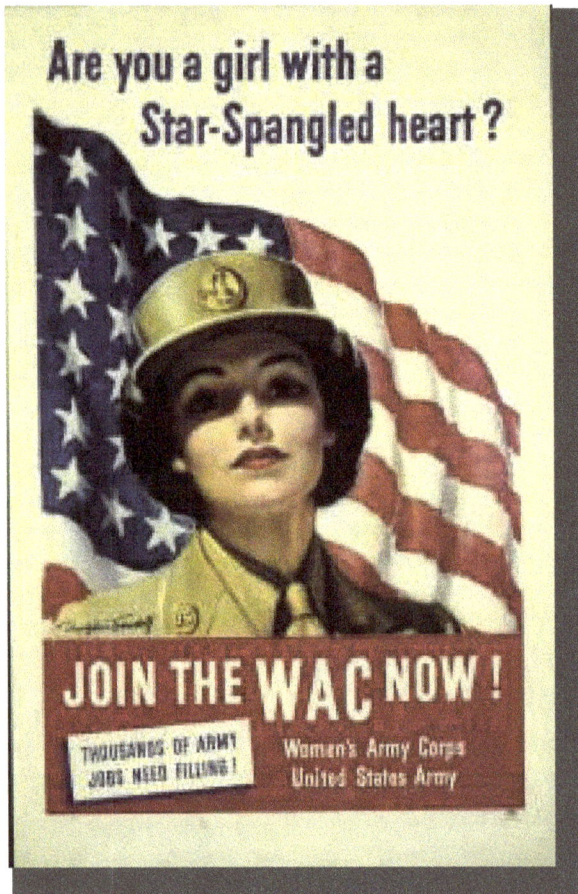

Women in the U.S. Army

1862—Clara Barton was appointed by Union Maj. Gen. Benjamin Butler as the "Lady in Charge" of the Army of the James.

1990—The largest call up of women since World War II, over 24,000 women served during Operation Desert Storm. **2015-** Army Directive 2016-01 opens more than 4,100 positions to women in the U.S Army Special Operations Command.

2016—Guidance to prepare for full integration of women.   All military occupations and positions become available to women, as long as they qualify and meet specific standards.

Women in the U.S. Coast Guard

1830's—Women were assigned as keepers in the lighthouse service.

1991—The Coast Guard established the women's advisory council.

2016—CDR Zeita Merchant became the first African-American woman to command a Prevention/Marine Safety unit.

Women in the U.S. Air force

1942—Women's Auxiliary Ferrying Squadron (WAFS) was formed.

2016—General Lori J. Robinson becomes first woman to lead a combatant command, US Northern Command and North American Aerospace Defense Command.

Women in the U.S. Marine Corps

1918—Private Opha Mae Johnson becomes the first woman to enlist in the Marine Corps Review.

1943—Private Lucille McClarren became the first enlisted woman.

2017—Combat roles opened for women. Women serve in 93 percent of all occupational fields and 62 percent of all billets. Women constitute 7.11% of the Corps end strength and are an integral part of the Marine Corps.

Women in the U.S. Navy

1862—Sisters of the Holy Cross served abroad USS Red Rover, the Navy's first hospital ship, joining a crew of 12 officers, 35 enlisted, and others supporting medical care. Red Rover remained the only hospital ship in the Navy until the Spanish-American War.

2014—Vice Adm. Jan. E. Tighe was appointed head of the U.S. Fleet Cyber Command and the U.S. 10th Fleet, making her the first female commander of a numbered fleet. Michelle Howard became the Navy's first female four-star admiral when she became vice-chief of naval operations.

Veterans

2017—Brigadier General (ret.), Loree Sutton, MD, was appointed commissioner for the New York City Department of Veterans Services (DVS).

New York was one of the first states to pass legislation giving women the right to vote in 1917, three years before the United States passed the 19th Amendment.

About the Author

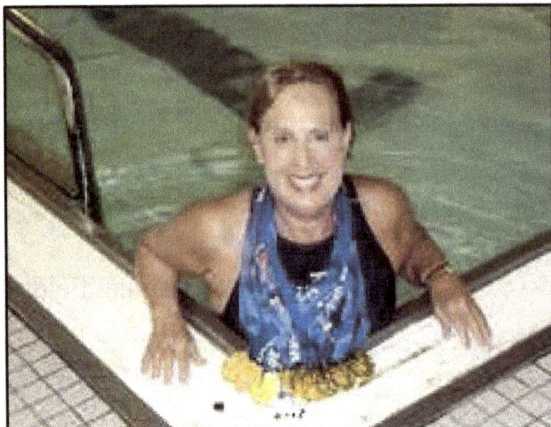

Dr. Jane Katz has taught thousands of students about the benefits of water fitness at the City University of New York (CUNY) since 1964, specifically for John Jay students since 1989. She is a Professor in the Department of Health and Physical Education as well as an aquatics innovator and author. Her primary expertise is educating the public on the benefits of aquatics for health and fitness.

As a member of the 1964 U.S. Synchronized Swimming Performance Team in Tokyo, Dr. Katz helped pioneer the acceptance of synchronized swimming as an Olympic event. Her achievements as a Master competitive, long distance, synchronized, and fin swimmer have earned her many All-American and World Master championships. At the Sydney Olympics in 2000 she was honored by Federation Internationale de Natation Amateur (FINA) with the Certificate of Merit for her 43 years of contribution to the sport of swimming. In 2014 she received the President's Council on Fitness, Sports & Nutrition Lifetime Achievement Award.

In 2004, for the second time she was voted Women's Swimming Coach of the year for the CUNY Division III schools. In 2007, Dr. Katz helped create the Kids Aquatic Re-Entry (KARE) Program, in cooperation with the New York City Department of Juvenile Justice to help troubled youth learn life's lessons poolside. She had also created Senior Exercise Programs geared towards aquatic fitness for older adults. Her latest splash is "W.E.T.s 4 VETS®" (Water Exercise Techniques for Veterans), a holistic program for returning veterans at John Jay College, to help them reintegrate into mainstream civilian life through Water Exercise Techniques.

Dr. Katz received the Outstanding Teacher Award for the 1999-2000 academic year at John Jay college. In 2010, Dr. Katz was the recipient of the Distinguished Faculty Award from John Jay College and in 2014 received the Distinguished Teaching Award sponsored by the John Jay College's Center for the Advancement of Teaching.

Dr. Katz grew up in the Lower East Side in New York City's Jewish community and she has not ignored her roots. She has been participating in the Maccabiah Games around the world since 1957. In 2011, she was the Team Captain for the USA Swim Team at the European Maccabiah Games in Vienna, Austria. In March 2011, Dr. Katz was inducted into the National Jewish Sports Hall of Fame and Museum In 2013, Dr. Katz swept the Maccabiah Games by winning eleven individual gold medals in her age group and an additional two medals in USA team relay events. Her latest splash was in Israel of July 2017 culminating in 60 years of Maccabiah Games.

In June of 2011, she was honored at the United Nations by the International Marathon Swimming Hall of Fame, given their Certificate of Merit Award, and three years later in Scotland was inducted into their Hall of Fame. In September 2012, she was inducted into the John Jay College Athletic Hall of Fame.

In 2013, Jane Katz was selected by Aquatics International as one of the 2013 "Power 25," a roundup of the most influential people in aquatics in the past 25 years, including Olympic superstars Michael Phelps, Janet Evans and Greg Lougains. The year 2014 marked both John Jay's and Dr. Katz's 50th anniversaries at CUNY. Dr. Katz has competed in the 2009, 2015, and 2017 National Senior Games.

Dr. Jane Katz is an accomplished writer with 14 books to her credit. Her first book published in 1981, Swimming for Total Fitness, was followed by videos, DVDs, CDs, newspaper and TV interviews, and numerous articles including Encyclopedia Britannica's "Take the Plunge: Swimming for Health," and "Aquatic Exercise."

List of Figures

APPENDICES

National Conference on Military Physical Fitness

NATIONAL CONFERENCE
ON MILITARY PHYSICAL FITNESS
1990

PROCEEDINGS REPORT

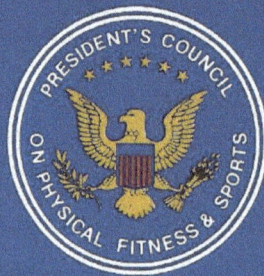

Presented by
The President's Council on Physical Fitness and Sports

U.S. DEPARTMENT OF HEALTH AND HUMAN SERVICES
Public Health Service

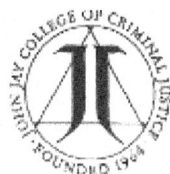

PERSPECTIVE: WATER EXERCISE — THE WAVE OF THE '90S

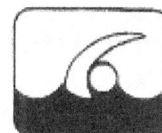

Jane Katz, Ed.D.

Dr. Katz is a recognized leader in the field of aquatics and physical fitness. She was a member of the Synchronized Swimming Performance Team in the 1964 Olympic Games. She holds numerous records and titles including the U.S. Masters' Solo Synchronized Swimming Champion since 1975, a Masters' All-American Swimming Champion since 1974, and a Long-Distance Champion since 1980. In 1989, she won five gold medals at the World Masters Swim Championships in Denmark, sweeping the freestyle events. Dr. Katz was chosen by The United States Jaycees as one of America's Ten Healthy American Fitness Leaders for 1987.

Swimming: An Essential Survival Technique

We have heard statistics that were alarming in terms of the number of members of the Armed Forces who don't swim, can't swim, or have not been exposed to any form of water fitness experience. As part of basic combat training, physical safety, and fitness, swimming is an essential survival technique. Not only are water exercises and swimming a necessary part of military physical fitness training, but also for other Uniformed Services such as the police and fire fighters, and those working in the substance abuse area. At the John Jay College of Criminal Justice at the City University of New York where I am a visiting professor, we are using water in all its forms to train these public servants to be physically fit in their professions, giving them also a lifetime of fitness and family activity.

The Ethnic Myth

I will put to rest the prevalent myth that ethnic people don't know how to swim or don't become good swimmers. For anyone who is not taught how to swim because of lack of opportunity or has never been near water, it is completely reasonable that he or she won't be able to swim. I've taught at Bronx Community College for the past 25 years, where the student body is 90 percent black and Hispanic, and everyone learned to swim. I also train with the City College Team in Harlem, which is composed almost entirely of black and Hispanic men and women of a wide age range. There is no problem, therefore, about ethnic capabilities, and this "old wives' tale" should be shed. If you are not exposed to water and not taught, it's not likely you are going to learn.

Water: Our Lifeline

We all come from a water environment. Two thirds of our body is water; three quarters of the earth is water. If we don't have water, we are in trouble; as for example, droughts in the land and dehydration of the body.

What I'd like to do now is take us through the wet world of water. [Slides were shown with text.]

Swimming for Play

Swimming is the most popular form of exercise in America. It is recreational. It is a family activity. It's lifetime. It is a superb conditioner of the body, mind, and spirit. Almost 100 million people use swimming and water exercise as their form of recreation. Thirty million people use lap swimming for fitness.

At the top of the pyramid are competitive swimmers and triathletes. For those in the military who compete at that level, the "X" factor is often swimming.

Water Exercise for Fitness

Water exercise is now expanding the horizons of fitness programs nationwide, civilian as well as military, where an astounding number have had no water training. Water exercise then becomes the entry level to developing fitness and safety, aiming toward swim skills and the cardiovascular benefits of an aerobic workout.

The broad base of the pyramid (the greatest number of participants) is immediately engaged in transferring skills from "sweats to wets" starting with the most familiar body movement—walking, that is—in water. With this very first step, the shape of a water workout begins to take form, namely warm-up, main set, and cool-down. This is the discipline practiced by the trained athlete. A workout should be between 30 and 45 minutes, with the warm-up using five to 10 minutes, main set 20 to 30 minutes for aerobic training effect, and the cool-down for about five minutes. The training effect occurs by applying the F.I.T. Principle of frequency, intensity, and time. A sample water exercise workout follows. For variety, use resistance devices such as a kickboard, which can also be used as a flotation support.

Exercise While Healing

Beyond the proven benefits of water exercise and swimming for survival and physical fitness, especially for members of the Military, there is the role of healing. Because the body weighs 10 percent of its weight in water, exercises that an injured or disabled person would find difficult to do on land are doable in water—thus participants build confidence and self-esteem from successfully having done a water exercise workout. ★

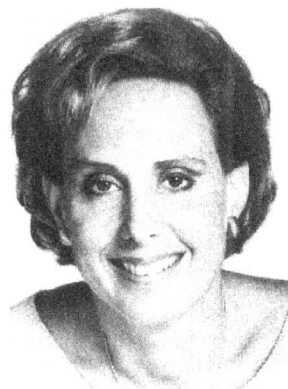

SAMPLE WATER EXERCISE PROGRAM

WARM-UP (5-10 minutes)

■ **Water walking.** Walk forward, backward, sideward, diagonally, in circles, etc.

■ **Water jogging.** Jog in all directions, using arms in opposition.

MAIN SET (20-30 minutes)

■ **Push-ups.** Stand with your body facing the wall and touching it, your hands on the pool's edge, shoulder-width apart. Straighten your elbows and lift your body out of the water.

■ **Torso rotations.** Place hands on hips. Turn your body to the right and return to starting position. Then turn to the left. For added resistance, extend arms sideward underwater, with palms facing down.

■ **Sit-ups.** Place your back against pool wall with arms outstretched and place hands on deck to support body in back float position. Bend your knees and bring them toward your chest. Then straighten them.

■ **Leg lifts.** Place your back against the pool wall with arms extended sideways on deck. Keeping legs straight, alternately lift them as close as possible to water's surface.

■ **Jumping jacks.** Stand with arms down at your sides. Turn your palms upward and bring them to water's edge as you separate your legs into a "V" position. Return to starting position by turning your palms downward and bringing them back to your sides as you bring legs together.

■ **Rope jump.** Simulate holding the handles of a jump rope with each hand at shoulder level with elbows touching the waist. As arms bring rope forward, knees bend and legs lift to clear rope. Continue jumping rope forward, then backward.

COOL-DOWN (5 minutes)

■ **Side-hip touch.** Stand next to pool wall an arm's distance away. Keeping your feet together, touch your hip to the wall, then stretch your hip as far as possible from the wall.

■ **Full body stretch.** Face the pool wall and hold onto edge with hands shoulder-width apart. Place feet against wall in a wide "V" position. Slowly flex and extend arms and legs to and from wall. For variation, alternately bend to each side.

Chart Your W.E.T.s 4 VETS Progress

DATE/TIME	AQUATIC SKILLS	WORKOUT LOCATION	PERSONAL COMMENTS/GOALS

Aquatic Workout Program

Personalize Your W.E.T.s 4 VETS®

Warm-up/Stretch (5 min.)   Comments:

Exercise Set 1 (5-8 min)

Exercise Set 2 (5-8 min)

Exercise Set 3 (5-8 min)

Cross Training Set 1 (5-8 min)

Cool down/Relaxation (5 min.)

Total Time (30-45 min.)

Emergency Contact Information

W.E.T.s 4 VETS
EMERGENCY CONTACT INFORMATION

NAME_____

ADDRESS_____

eMAIL_____

PHONE_____

EMERGENCY CONTACT

Name_____ Relationship_____

Address_____

Phone_____

SIGN IN SHEET

Event _____   Date _____

#	First Name	Last Name
1		
2		
3		
4		
5		
6		
7		
8		
9		
10		
11		
12		
13		
14		

Sample Medical Waiver

Participating in physical activities such as swimming is a vigorous activity and you are doing so AT YOUR OWN RISK. A medical evaluation is strongly recommended. If you have any health considerations, please inform your instructor.

Last Name	First Name	Date

THR Chart

Date	Activity W.E.T.s 4 VETS	Warm-Up	Main Set	Cool Down	Comments
Today	*Stretch*				

Dr. J's Tips for Swimmers

1. Get a medical check-up before beginning any physical exercise program.

2. Swim with a buddy.

   a. Swim in a supervised area with a lifeguard on duty.

   b. Never swim alone.

3. Begin slowly and progress steadily toward a goal.

   a. If you feel tired or persistent pain, stop.

   b. Listen to your body.

   c. Chart/record your progress

4. Follow the rules of the pool, especially safety regulations. Please be considerate of others.

5. When you swim in a lap lane, circle counterclockwise by staying to the right.

   a. To pass someone, slow down and wait for the wall. Most swimmers when asked will yielded the lane, so say thank you.

   b. An alternate strategy is to wait at the wall for the slow swimmer then begin your laps.

6. Warm-up before your main swim set and cool-down afterwards for about 5 minutes.

7. Change up your workout by using swim equipment for drills and/or water exercises.

8. At an outdoor pool, leave the water when requested by lifeguards in anticipation of lightning.

9. Diving into the water is prohibited at most pools now. Please follow the local pool's rules.

10. Wear a comfortable suit, goggles, swim cap, and for most pools bring a towel and padlock.

Swim Notes:

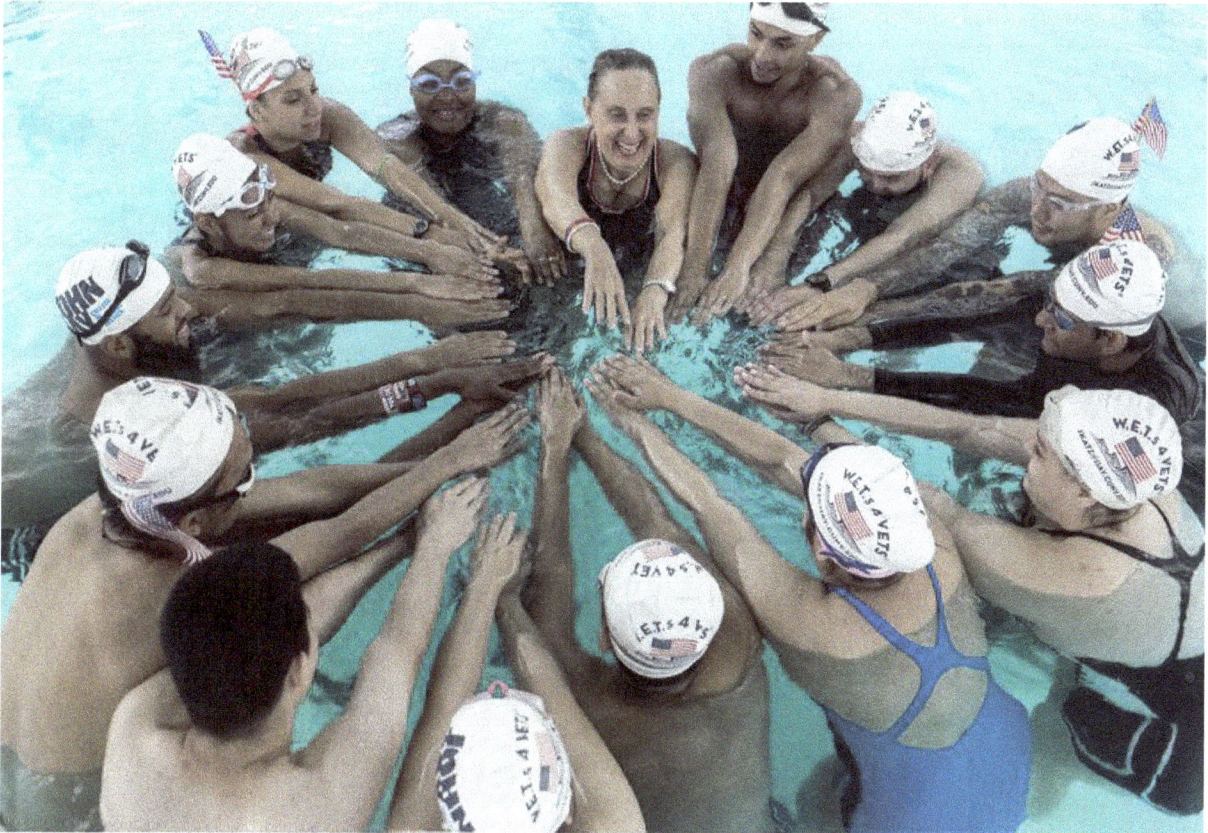

A group of veterans and students at John Jay College of Criminal Justice gathers in a circle during a "WETs 4 Vets" class. Will Glaser/The New York Times

www.ingramcontent.com/pod-product-compliance
Lightning Source LLC
Chambersburg PA
CBHW081650270326
41933CB00018B/3418

9 781734 046304